CHRONIC FATIGUE SYNDROME
A.I.D.S &
IMMUNE DYSFUNCTION
DISEASE

THE CAUSE
AND THE CURE

Suzann Marie Angelus

Hypnotherapist   Sound Researcher

Symbolic Productions
Moraga, California

Chronic Fatigue Syndrome, A.I.D.S., and Immune
Dysfunction Disease: The Cause and The Cure

Cover Design & Illustration: Lightbourne Images, Ashland, Oregon ©1994
Book Design and Copy Layout: Carol Hansen, Concord, CA
Graphic Design: Tim Manning, Pleasant Hill, CA
Indexing: Nancy Freedom, Oakland, CA

Library of Congress Catalog Card Number: 94-66071

Publisher's Cataloging in Publication
(Prepared by Quality Books Inc.)

Angelus, Suzann Marie,
    Chronic fatigue syndrome, A.I.D.s. & immune dysfunction disease
: the cause and the cure / by Suzann Marie Angelus.

    p. cm.
    Includes bibliographical references and index.
    ISBN 0-9640559-9-6

    1. Chronic fatigue syndrome. 2. AIDS (Disease) 3. Immune
system—Diseases. I. Title. II. Title: Chronic fatigue syndrome,
AIDS and immune dysfunction disease.

RB150.F37A54 1994   616.9'25
                                           QBI94-557

First Edition
Printed in the United States of America

I dedicate this book to my three boys
in the hope that they will some day
understand my ordeal.
and the love I have for them.

and

To my beloved Angelo. whose love and
support has kept me moving forward
even in times of great despair...

and

To all those who suffer from CFIDS
or other immune dysfunction...
I pray that this book offers you hope.

Finally. I offer a prayer for all humanity...

Father-Mother God.
I pray that the information contained in this book
will bring about the dawning of a new consciousness.
not only in medicinebut in politics as well.
I pray that those who have brought this planet
and all lifeforms on it
to the brink of destruction.
will be removed and replaced by a higher consciousness.
I pray that the days of a consciousness fear and war
be replaced by a consciousness of love
and concern for the earth and all of its inhabitants.
May we unite in one body and one voice
for the survival of the earth.
May reverence for the Great Mother Earth
and her natural laws be restored.

CONTENTS

i

PART 3

SOURCES OF CONTAMINATION 117

PART 4

HELP IF YOU HAVE CHRONIC FATIGUE SYNDROME 133

INTRODUCTION

Estimates of those suffering with Chronic Fatigue Syndrome in the U.S. run as high as 10 million, depending upon who you believe. The U.S. Health Department and Center for Disease Control don't seem to take CFIDS very seriously. In spite of this lack of interest, more and more people are coming down with the symptoms. Have you noticed that prescription medicines used to control yeast and candida infections are now available over the counter? Could it be because there is an epidemic of chronic yeast infections? Today, thousands of people find themselves unable to work or function at a meaningful level. Forced to give up work, most watch in quiet desperation as their life's work slips through their fingers. This includes financial security, mates, children, friends and other loved ones. The medical community offers little hope. Many hospitals and medical plans refuse to treat CFIDS. Many CFIDS sufferers commit suicide, or attempt it.

As figures climb in other countries, CFIDS is taken more seriously. A world problem affecting millions and millions of people, this is only the beginning. More and more people will manifest symptoms, waste away, and slowly die. How do I know this for a fact? I state this as a fact because I know what is causing Chronic Fatigue Syndrome.

Citizens of the world, listen up: there is no place to hide. This disease will not go away by itself. It is the same disease killing birds, fish, deer, dolphins, mammals and all creatures who call planet earth home. Perhaps it has taken longer to manifest in humans because we are larger and our bodies can tolerate more chemicals before it breaks down. Chronic

v

Fatigue Syndrome is a disease caused by chemical pollution, radiation and pesticides. CFIDS is a disease of nuclear war, radiation, and nerve gas chemicals. It is the end result of a world wide philosophy of industrialization and production of synthetic chemicals. It is the end result of fear and the war mentality that has existed on earth for thousands of years. It is the result of the" power and control" philosophy of the patriarchal society which pervades our world. It is the result of a world out of touch with nature and natural laws.

I speak from my own personal experience. Reduced to an invalid for twelve years of my life, I refused to accept the fact that there was no cure. Refusing to die, I left no stone unturned to find the cause and to heal myself. I was willing to explore new ideas and new ways of healing. I stretched myself into the past to regain information and knowledge and bring that knowledge into the present. I share my journey here in the hopes that this information will assist others in regaining their health.

The world must change if we are to survive. We must unite and focus to clean up the mess we have created here. The earth can be saved. The people can be saved as well.

My process has worked for others as well. Considered unconventional by the medical community and those of a conservative nature, I am sure that it will be awhile before it is widely embraced and accepted. My cure involves no drugs, radiation, or surgery. This healing process involves an abundant, natural food that is readily available on the planet, along with hypnosis to release genetic information encoded in the electromagnetic energy of the subtle bodies which effect the DNA. I feel confident that it can help many who are ready to leave this disorder behind and move forward with life.

I am not a doctor, nor trained in any traditional scientific or medical disciplines. I might best be described as a meta-physician or mystic. In the process of healing myself, I have recovered much ancient knowledge involving the process of healing the physical through working with the subtle bodies. I share that knowledge with you in a way that I hope you will be able to understand.

PART 1

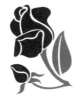

My Twelve Year
Personal Experience
with
Chronic Fatigue Syndrome.

PART I

MY TWELVE YEAR PERSONAL EXPERIENCE WITH CFIDS

First, let me say that I never thought I would be writing a book, any book, much less one on the subject of Chronic Fatigue Syndrome. However, much has changed in my life. My life before Chronic Fatigue somehow seems so far away; it sometimes feels like a past life memory. Perhaps that is another one of the tolls this disease has exacted from me.

The fact that I am able to comprehensively write and organize my thoughts is a major accomplishment in itself. Afflicted with the typical loss of memory and concentration that affects most CFIDS (Chronic Fatigue Immune Dysfunction Syndrome) victims, this is a feat I thought I would never perform again in my life. To me, it is another indication that I am well and regaining my full mental capacity after many years of not having important parts functioning and available to me.

This is my story. Unlike most CFIDS sufferers, it is a triumphant one. I feel compelled to share it with others and offer them hope that they, too, can recover from this devastating disability. I hope that the information that I have uncovered that has led to my recovery will assist others to do the same. I have basically tried to stick to the facts, and share information. I am not sure that I have the capacity to put into words the emotional and psychological impact this disease has had on my life. I can fairly accurately measure the financial one. I can even

3

attempt in some way to communicate to you the physical impact, as I can talk about symptoms and loss of function. The impossible part is the psychological and emotional impact.

There are no words to express the years of despair, confusion, pain, ridicule, abandonment, misunderstanding and lack of support that one feels as a victim of this disorder. I felt deserted and abandoned by my family who had no way of understanding what I was going through. Because I was unable to obtain a medical diagnosis, I was ridiculed and put down by my husband and loved ones. I was ridiculed by my doctors who seemed to get great satisfaction out of telling me I was perfectly healthy. No one could hear me or would hear me.

Later, I was to be labeled as someone who did not have to work, or was looking for an excuse not to work. I was even ridiculed by the psychologists and counselors I sought out for advice and support. I have been laughed at, told I was crazy, and discredited. Despite everything, I kept going. Not always sure what it was I was looking for, I kept moving forward in a direction that would one day bring me out the other side.

Once I made the decision to write this book, I attended a workshop on self publishing. It was very comprehensive and inspired me to move forward. One of the first things that I learned about writing a book was to do market research on other books currently available on the subject. That sounded like a reasonable place to start, so I went off to the book store to check out the subject of Chronic Fatigue Syndrome. Keep in mind, most of my personal research was done in San Rafael, California, and Maui, totally without contact with other researchers. I was very pleasantly surprised when many of the books I found on CFIDS indicated almost identical facts, symptoms, and conclusions about the disease. This made me feel even more confident that I have information to offer to the millions of people in the world who suffer from this disorder. The one thing that the books on CFIDS could not offer was a cause. They could only speculate that the cause would be discovered soon.

So, I write this book to share with you the cause of CFIDS, AIDS and other immune dysfunction diseases. I can even tell you a lot more than is currently known about the cause of viruses and other "overgrowth". I will share with you a lot of information you might have trouble believing or understanding. However, knowing the cause is a long way from finding the cure. As you will see, there is no easy cure for this disease.

There will be no miracle drug or miracle cure. Many will die after years of tremendous personal suffering, psychological as well as physical. Some will survive. I wish I could wave a magic wand and offer a cure for all. At best, it will be a slow process to recovery. But I can offer you hope. I have survived to tell the story and am recovering my full abilities. I have helped others who are recovering. Many cannot afford my services. Some will not believe what I have to say. Still others will not want to believe what I have to say. I can only say in truth, "Look at me, I have been to the bottom with this disease, and I have recovered." What I have to share with you may help you as well. I am willing to work with those who are serious about being cured. By serious, I mean that you may have to make lifestyle changes on many levels, but it's not impossible and can be done. I am limited in what I can do for others, as I am not a doctor. I am not trained in the medical sciences, but I know that what I have done for myself will work for others as well. I am here to share this information with all those who will listen.

MY BACKGROUND

I always considered myself a pretty "typical" person. By that I mean that there is nothing really outstanding about me that would distinguish my life from most Americans.

I was born in Louisville, Kentucky, on March 16, 1943. I was raised in a well meaning but typically dysfunctional family that we hear a lot about today. My father was in the Navy when I was born, where he taught aircraft mechanics. Later, he worked as an aircraft mechanic and serviced planes at Louisville Flying Service.

He was a very handsome man who was confused and angry. He worked very hard to support a wife and five kids, but did not seem to know what to do with them. I remember him as an angry, controlling person who made life miserable for most of us. I was absolutely terrified of my father. He prided himself on "making us walk the chalkline" and seemed to think that if we were potty trained and appropriately disciplined he was successful as a father.

6

There was no love or kindness in the family. The atmosphere was more like the "reign of terror". There were rules for everything, and we (my sisters and brother) spent most of the time tiptoeing around, hoping not to disturb or awaken the sleeping giant. I developed a tremendous sense of guilt or wrong doing, always feeling that I had done something wrong, or might do something wrong which would incur the wrath of my father. My father would sit in his chair in the living room for days on end, angry at us, but unable to communicate why he was angry. We lived daily with the anxiety of knowing that we had done something wrong, but not understanding what.

Later, as I grew up, I would learn that he was an alcoholic. Perhaps that explains a lot. I am not sure. Later in life, he developed a strange and mysterious disease that attacked his nervous system and brain and left him a vegetable for the last 15 years of his life. Under constant medical care, the doctors were baffled as to the source of his affliction.

As I look back now, I have the greatest sympathy for my mother. My father controlled everything, even her. He had the money and the car. I remember that he would take her to the grocery store and wait in the car while she would shop. No matter how fast she would shop, she always took too long. He would be angry and irritated as he went into the grocery store to write the check. She was not allowed to sign checks or have any money of her own. Years later, I was to learn that he lied to her for years, telling her that the insurance would not cover her so she could not drive. One of my first jobs was working for an independent insurance agent. Imagine my surprise when I learned this was not true! His attitude was to keep her at home with no money, or car, or friends. She could not even attend church functions without his permission.

During the summer of 1957, we moved to Alaska. My father took a job with the Federal Aviation Agency. The job description was in Anchorage, Alaska. As we did research on Alaska, we found that there were lots of bars, airplanes and snow. Rightly so, we thought we were moving to the ends of the earth. This was the wild west, the new frontier: a land of new adventure and a promise of more money.

Needless to say, from the time I was very young, I plotted for the day of my escape. I wanted to be grown up so that I could get out of there. I got a full time job babysitting during the summer as soon as I was old enough. I saved my money carefully until I could afford a car. Then, I was on the road to independence.

I matured early. I sometimes think that I was born into this world 5'8" tall. I sprouted up there during my pre-teens. This left me taller than any of the boys in school. Living in Alaska, which was still the "Last Frontier", I soon found that I was in demand by older men. Keep in mind that men outnumbered women 10 to 1 in Alaska in the 1960's. By the time I was 17, I was dating my future husband. I met my husband of 20 years during the summer between my junior and senior year of high school.

I had no problem passing for 21 and enjoyed going

out to supper clubs where we could ballroom dance. I never really liked to drink alcohol. I did not like the taste. But there was something more to it. Everyone else was getting relaxed and free, but all I ever experienced was tension. The more I drank, the more sober and tense I became. I would get headaches. Martinis were the popular thing to drink. My future husband and all his friends drank them. They tasted like gasoline to me. However, I did not want to order coke, thinking it would be a give away that I was underage, so I would order a martini and sip on it all night long. I never did develop a taste for alcohol. Over time, I settled for a glass of wine or two.

I was married at age 20. My husband was born and raised in Alaska to an old pioneering family. At the time we were married he was 31 years old and was very successful at his profession. We began raising a family right away. Between babies I would take college classes at the local university. The early years were busy and happy ones. Besides birthing three children in five years, we skied, played tennis, and led a very active social life typical of a professional person. This included cocktail parties, service organizations, professional conventions, and dinner parties. My husband was interested in politics and we had many politician friends. Life was busy, and I was happy.

My days were busy keeping house and taking care of babies. I really loved cooking. I especially loved baking cookies, breads, and sweet things for the kids. Those were busy years. I seemed happy. I longed to be closer to my husband. He was nice and took good care of me, and we had all the things that money and success could bring.

However, I longed for intimacy with him. I wanted to be able to share my thoughts and feelings with him. He did not seem to be able to do this. He seemed embarrassed about his feelings, unable to communicate with me on any level except intellectually. He seemed content with our life the way it was. His work kept him preoccupied. He read a lot when he was not working. He had no real interest or aptitude for helping around the house.

I did not feel much either. I wanted to feel things, and wanted to share. However, I found that I did not have feelings like other people. At a young age, I noticed I was insensitive to hot sensations. I noticed other people's reactions to burns or hot liquid spills. They seemed to experience a lot of pain. That was not my case however. My nervous system was different. Although I felt burns, I did not seem to be as sensitive to pain. I wondered what could be different about my nervous system.

I was the ultimate mother. I took care of my husband and took care of things. As long as his clothes were clean, his suits pressed for work, his house clean and his meals on time, he was content.

When the children were young, I kept busy mothering everyone. As the children were enrolled in school. I began to look forward to doing other things. I wanted to go back to school. I felt unfulfilled. There was something missing in all of this, some deep aching feeling for love and intimacy.

CRISIS OF THE THIRTIES - 1970'S

When my thirties arrived, I was in crisis. I was feeling the need to grow up and make some changes in my life. I felt that everything was fine as long as I minded like a good wife and did what I was supposed to do. Deep inside I felt like my husband was my father, and I was a little girl, minding her Daddy, afraid to strike out on her own. I needed to grow up and find out who I was. This is when my marriage started to fall apart. My husband was always very jealous of other men. In the early days of courting, I was not introduced to his single friends out of fear that they might want to date me. By the time I was thirty, I was in need of some freedom. My husband, threatened by the idea of my being in the outside world, wanted to have more babies to keep me at home. That was the last thing I needed.

By now, I was on birth control. This was a tense issue with us. My husband wanted more babies. I knew for certain I did not. In 1965, I had experienced a placenta praevia condition with the birth of my youngest boy. During the emergency Cesarean Section that followed, I left my body and went through the light tunnel into the other side. What a profound experience it was! There were many bright light beings who seemed to know me and communicated their happiness in my presence there. I felt so wonderful. There was so much love in this place. I was ready to stay. I did not want to leave this love. I had never experienced this feeling in my life on earth.

Suddenly, I found myself in a meeting with other beings in authority. I was told that I could not stay. I had to return to earth and this human body because I had work to do. There was not time for me to reincarnate and start over. I must return now. Before I could voice my objections, I found my consciousness on the ceiling of the recovery room looking down at my body. I could clearly see the nurse and my husband standing by my side. Quickly, I slipped into my body, and woke up. Then I proceeded to throw up as this had been an emergency procedure and the meatloaf sandwich I had for lunch was on its way out.

The baby was fine, and I would recover. We both received several blood transfusions during the ordeal, a fact that I feel contributed greatly to our loss of health years later. My son, Tim, has experienced immune dysfunction parallel to mine. Today, I definitely feel that one or both of us received tainted blood, and that this was the initial source of the Chronic Fatigue Syndrome. If it were not the sole cause, it contributed greatly. Although I did not develop AIDS, I am totally convinced that I did eventually develop HTLV 1 & 2 viruses which are in the same family as AIDS and will cause leukemia.

I knew then that I would not have more children. I did not consciously know why. I suggested to my husband that if he wanted more children, we could adopt them. He would not consider that possibility.

When I tried to communicate my death experience, he laughed and told me that I was hallucinating under the anesthesia. I knew differently. It was much later that the books on life after death and the movie, "Resurrection", confirmed my experience as valid.

The distance between us widened. I was drawn to yoga and metaphysics. He would accuse me of deliberately embracing beliefs and ideas that would anger him. I tried to get him into counseling. He was not interested.

I went to counseling. I decided that I needed to prove to myself that I could do something besides have babies and keep house. I started a retail business. That kept me very busy. However, my husband got more threatened. He would vacillate between being very happy and excited for me when he was sober and threatening me when he was drunk. I hated the drinking. I was afraid of the person who came to life from the alcohol. There was so much anger and irrational thinking. I begged him to get help.

We grew further and further apart. He was out a lot "drinking with the boys". He would come home drunk and nasty. I begged him to do something about his drinking problem. He was in denial and not interested. I was the only one with problems, not him. I wanted to make changes in our life. Although he insisted that he was happy, I was convinced that he was in a lot of pain. Out of fear of change, he wanted to keep things just as they were. My job was to have babies, and take care of the family and house. I spent a lot of time beating myself up emotionally, trying to make myself fit into this narrow role which was defined for me. I felt guilty that I needed more. I wanted fulfillment in my life. There was this huge empty ache inside. Why was I not happy? I had everything in the world that should make me happy. At least that was what

I had been led to believe. I felt trapped and stifled. I needed more.

I started planning for the day when I would ask for a divorce. To be a mother with three young boys with no job experience was an overwhelming thought for me. I did not want to break up the family while the boys were so young. I did not want my children to go through the heartbreak of a divorce. Perhaps I could delay this for a time. I was also concerned about my safety. My husband was not going to let go of me and his family without a fight.

I became more and more independent. We drifted further and further apart. We took separate vacations. I sold the business I had started and became a real estate agent, then a broker. Later, I was to have my own company. I made decisions that involved a lot of money. Although it was stressful at times, I was very good at it. I had good intuitions about real estate investments. I had invested our money and bought property throughout our marriage. My timing was good. During the following years, I was to make a lot of money in the real estate business. Much later, I was very grateful for the money, as I was able to support myself during the years I could not work. I became absorbed in my work.

My health started downhill. I developed acute allergies to household dust and cigarette smoke. I was not able to vacuum or dust my own house. The children were allergic to dust as well. Suddenly, I was unable to tolerate cigarette smoke of any kind. I never smoked myself. The only time I was exposed was in restaurants, nightclubs, and public places. I stopped going out to these places. About the same time, I found myself unable to sleep at night. That seemed understandable considering the circumstances.

I went into marriage counseling. My husband refused. My doctor put me on Valium. Reading statistics on the number of women on tranquilizers, it bothered me a lot to think I was joining these statistics. At that time, I could do nothing about it.

Then the infections started. At first it was sinus infections which progressed into bladder and kidney infections. Still later, it was vaginal infections. I was on antibiotics for almost a year solid. Besides bacterial infections, I now had to contend with yeast infections. It was a constant problem. My doctor did not seem to be alarmed. I was alarmed, however. It seemed that every time I ate something sweet, I would get an infection which seemed to take turns popping out in different organs.

I wore an IUD. If my memory serves me right, it was called a Lippy's Loop and made out of copper. My doctor did not think this was contributing to the problem. I was reassured that it was very safe. Because CFIDS was to hit women so hard, I wondered later if there was a relationship between CFIDS and women who wore IUDs. That would be a very interesting statistic to pursue sometime.

Whatever was happening to me seemed overwhelming. I suddenly developed problems with my shoulders, diagnosed as scapulary fibrosis. I took up swimming in order to relieve the pain caused by the muscles in my neck and shoulders locking up. Swimming was painful, as the process of moving the arms would force my neck out of place and I would have to have chiropractic adjustments. The muscles along the spine were very tight. They would lockup and would not release. The pain was similar to a "charley horse". I would walk around for days or weeks with a terrible pain. Sometimes it felt like my eyes were going to pop out of my head. Also, I was having problems with spastic colon. My doctor told me that it was stress related. I could believe that. I felt really stressed out. Something was really wrong with my health. I had always been very athletic and healthy. This was new for me.

My dog came down with spastic colon about the same time. It did not take long for him to develop into colitis and Nugget died. Golden Nugget was a beautiful golden retriever. He was young and frisky and needed lots of affection. Unfortunately, he was often too frisky with the children and his playful interludes would end with him being sent outside to the dog pen. He would knock them over with his wagging tail, or nip at them playfully. When the tears would start, playtime would end. He was lots of fun in the outdoors, and loved going off into the woods with us hiking and camping.

He seemed very young to get colitis. If my memory is right, Nugget was only 4-5 years old. Deep inside, I felt that he did not get enough affection. My days were busy with the three boys and keeping up the house. I did not have much time left over to spend with the dog. I was deeply saddened at his death. It seems strange to me now that my dog and I came down with the same disease.

With the knowledge that I have today about CFIDS, I would look for some common source of contamination. I would definitely test the water. Most certainly I would test the soil for radiation or other toxic materials. CFIDS often passes through family members and household pets. Although I state in my lectures that I feel that CFIDS is a communicable disease and that the viruses can be passed through the same avenues as AIDS or any other virus, I had forgotten about Nugget until I started writing this book. In this type of situation, I would look deeper than a virus, I would look for a common source of radiation exposure or other toxic chemicals.

My teeth started breaking. I remember the first time it happened. I crunched down on a piece of peanut brittle during a Christmas party. Snap. I felt my back molar break in two. That was just the beginning. There would be many more to come. I found out much later that the broken teeth had to do with lack of calcium in my body.

I was born with some deformed vertebrae in my lower back and a partial fusion. Up until now, it had never really bothered me. With the onset of the scapulary fibrosis, and muscle cramps, my spine needed lots of attention. I started regular chiropractic visits. The cramping muscles were pulling the vertebrae out of alignment. I was developing spurs along my spine.

I developed digestive problems. After eating any kind of food, I would develop a smelly gas. Later I was to learn that this was a symptom of candida overgrowth in the intestinal tract.

I spent thousands and thousands of dollars during a two to three year period having blood tests done and trying to convince my doctor that there was something wrong with me. This doctor also treated my father who had major problems going on. As I mentioned earlier, my father developed some major brain and nervous system disorder that left him a vegetable for at least 15 years. I was beginning to see some parallel with my father's early symptoms and my own. When I raised this point to my doctor, he became very defensive and hostile. After that, it was like he was out to prove me wrong. He just kept reassuring me that there was absolutely nothing wrong. I was in perfect health. Perhaps I was stressed out, and needed to make some decisions about my life.

I agreed with him on that. I could not put off my decisions for a divorce much longer. The situation was causing me a lot of stress. But there was more to this than that. Deep down inside, I was convinced there was some physical cause of this stress. One could not feel like I did and not have physical symptoms. I simply would not believe that there was nothing physically wrong.

I was very upset, however, with my doctor's attitude. Suddenly, he had a closed mind. There would be no convincing him of anything. I decided to get another opinion, and made an appointment to see another internist in the clinic. Much to my surprise, this doctor had blackballed me in the clinic and no one would see me. What a shock!

Not easily rebuffed, I made an appointment with an internist at another clinic and went in for another opinion. When the blood tests came back, I was confronted with a very similar situation. Basically, I was a over-reactive female who suffered from PMS. Only this doctor took things a step further and told me to flush all my vitamins down the toilet as they did absolutely no good. To think that I paid money for this advice!

Thus began several frustrating and heartbreaking years of doctors and rebuffs. At one point, I was so frustrated that I made an appointment at the Mason Clinic in Seattle and flew out with my records. I took along the hospital records from my last childbirth. Something told me even then that there was some key here. I expected the doctors to find it. I was disappointed. Rebuffed again, I was made to feel that I was an impulsive female who would not take the sound advice given to her by well qualified physicians. My relationship with doctors and traditional medicine was becoming very strained. I knew I was not crazy. I knew something was very wrong. Why would no one listen to me?

I had to believe the blood test. The only experience of medicine that I had to date was traditional medicine. Although I could not imagine that what was going on in my body was strictly stress related, I had to believe those blood tests that kept saying there was nothing wrong with me. Maybe I was going crazy.

There was no support at home, either. Besides everything else, my husband was not at all supportive about my illness. It was all very black and white to him. The doctors were right. I was making all of this up. There was nothing wrong with me. I just needed to get ahold of myself. I was spending all this money on doctors and psychologists because it was the fashionable thing to do.

The day of separation from my husband finally came. Actually, he asked for a divorce one night after being out drinking with some friends. I was somewhat relieved and began making plans to move. At last, the step had to be taken. By now, I was having a lot of difficulty thinking and acting rationally. I could not concentrate on anything for very long. I had lost my ability to read and remember what I had just read. He went off to New York on business. Upon his return he announced that it was all a big mistake and that he did not want a divorce. I told him that there was no turning back. I had seen an attorney while he was away. Neither one of us was happy. I was not going to reconsider. He was very angry about my reply and informed me that he would not cooperate. I was going to have to move out of the house and away from the children, as he would not move out until the courts pronounced us divorced.

I think that this was the first time in my life that I had the courage to stand up to him and say "no". I was in a lot of pain and confusion. I just wanted some peace in my life. This situation needed to change. I was afraid of what was happening to me. My life was falling apart on all levels. No one would support me. I was better off alone.

As I look back now upon my marriage, I wonder just how much of the breakup could be contributed to the CFIDS. Perhaps I will never know the answer to that question. I realize that the alcohol was a major contribution. In the years to follow, I have learned much about co-addictive relationships and substance abuse. My husband's childhood and upbringing was not a happy one either. There were a lot of deep issues that needed to be addressed. Perhaps I could have been more helpful. As I learn more and more about the deep level of dysfunction in our society, I understand why couples cannot stay together. We are all deeply wounded. Few have the skills to heal themselves, much less assist others.

By this time, I was in survival mode, and sinking very fast. It had been just about ten years after the blood transfusion that my health began to fall apart. Within five years, my marriage, my business and my whole life collapsed.

I packed and moved in with a friend. I was so sick by then that I felt like a zombie most of the time. By now, I could not read or concentrate, finding myself unable to remember the last sentence I just read. My brain was in a fog all the time. My physical body was in a lot of pain. I had just wanted a place to sleep and rest. Something was very wrong with my nervous system.

My personality changed. There were deep psychological issues surfacing. There had been no sex in our marriage for the last seven years, and I was attracted to other men. I was in my sexual prime. I decided to have an affair. Intellectually, it seemed an "OK" thing to do. I felt awful. I hated sneaking around. I was overwhelmed with incredible guilt. The movies made it look very glamorous. I did not like myself very much. I seemed addicted to this person who mistreated me. When I started dating other men I noticed a definite pattern; I kept drawing into my life abusive, violent, unfeeling men. This alarmed me a great deal.

Where were all the loving men? I had single girl friends who could go out dancing or go to workshops and meet really nice men. That was not the case for me. I seemed to attract men who wanted to play around, had addictions, were abusive, and wanted to live off me. I call this type of personality "users and abusers".

Since I had little dating experience before I was married, finding myself suddenly single was a little overwhelming. Not only did I have to deal with the strict, unhappy, abusive childhood, I was also raised Catholic and spent 8 years in a Catholic school. Everything seemed to be a sin. It seemed to me that all my life, some authority figure was telling me what to do and how to do it. Someone was there to condemn me for whatever I did. I needed to find out what I believed in myself. I went through my own rebellion stage. I threw out all the "shoulds" and "musts" and started over. I seemed lost and out of control. Something inside of me wanted a man to be there and take care of me. I was embarrassed to be a woman alone in a restaurant or bar. Men came on to me. I had some romantic idea that I was going to meet my prince charming and fall in love. Everything would be just great. That was not the case. I realized that there was a real conflict going on inside. I did not understand it. I did not understand this person inside who was so out of control. I eventually realized that I needed help. I could get seriously hurt. I stopped dating and started doing inner work to find out why this was happening.

Today, I understand more about the psychological

impact that abuse and violence has on people. I am sure that was part of what I went through. However, I also feel that some of what I experienced was a result of the conditions in my body caused by a swollen and infected brain. Although I cannot prove it by conventional means, I am totally convinced that this condition was brought on by a blood transfusion I received at the birth of my youngest son. Perhaps I was possessed. I do not know for sure. As I look back on my life, this period was, without question, the most confusing and painful part of my life. I have had some difficulty loving and accepting this confused person. I wish sometimes that this period had never happened. However, I have come to trust in God. I have come to believe that everything that happens to you is an opportunity to grow. We all fall down at times; we all make mistakes. It is what one does with those mistakes that counts. This was just one phase of my life that was changed by Chronic Fatigue Syndrome. There were many other aspects that changed as well.

There is a law in the universe that "Like Attracts Like". In other words, if you have certain vibrations in your energy field, they will send out a signal that will attract others into your space with a similar vibration. If you have a lot of repressed anger, you will draw angry people into your life. Certain drugs or toxic chemicals in your body will draw people into your life with similar drugs or chemicals. This is why it is so difficult for a person with an addiction to make changes. The chemical substances leave residues in the body that feed the desire for more. They also affect the brain, nervous system and personality of that person, and contribute greatly to the pattern of addiction. One needs to look further into the victims for certain toxic chemical residues. When they are eliminated from the body, that person can truly begin to make changes and other people's reactions to them will change as well.

I know this from my own personal experience. I was to eventually learn that when I received tainted blood in a transfusion, the people and situations in my life changed almost immediately. As long as there were drugs and other extremely toxic chemicals in my body, I was constantly drawing people into my life with similar chemical vibrations in their system. It took me many years to figure this one out, but my life has changed since I discovered the presence of these drugs and eliminated them from my energy field with "sound". Today, I am with one of the most loving men I have ever met. Once again, I have supportive people in my life.

INTRODUCTION TO
ALTERNATIVE MEDICINE

We all meet people in our lives that are responsible for profound changes. Often they will show up at a time of great crisis to teach us new skills and help us open new doorways. Jai Inder was just such a person to me.

As I look back today I cannot remember how we met, but I am thankful that our paths crossed when they did. A busy chiropractor today, Jai was a massage therapist who ran a holistic healing center in Anchorage. She used all kinds of skills and knowledge to help me open to a new way of healing and looking at health. She recognized the great pain and suffering I was experiencing and recommended that I have a hair analysis done to determine if I was deficient in vitamins and minerals. She used kiniesology to help determine correct dosages. She educated me on massage and diet.

Finally, sensing the seriousness of my condition, she recommended that I have a psychic medical reading. I was from a very, very straight, traditional background and was not sure I even knew what a psychic was. However, I was desperate and made an appointment to see this man. I became very, very thankful when he began rattling off this long list of dysfunctional things in my body. First, he said that I had major digestive problems: I was not digesting my food. Grains were turning into alcohol in my intestines. I needed digestive enzymes with my meals. I suffered from food poisoning. I had no calcium in my body. I was suffering from a prolapsed colon. I had parasites. He also said that I suffered from systemic candida and fungus overgrowth as well as systemic blood staph infection. Finally, he said that I had pre-cancerous cells in my small intestine, and suggested that I take liquid colloidal minerals that would flush them out.

I was somewhat relieved that someone finally agreed with me that I was not in good health. Here was a confirmation of my feelings that something was very wrong in my body. You can imagine the questions in my mind. I had spent thousands of dollars on traditional medicine, only to be told that there was nothing wrong with me. Then, I found out from a psychic that I was really quite sick. He referred me to a medical doctor who treated candida and could help with some of the other problems.

The mention of cancer brought real fear into me. However, there was a part of me that felt my condition was serious enough to be cancer. At least a cancer diagnosis would give me a name for my ailment. We could begin treating something. I was encouraged. So, I made an appointment to see this doctor and he began to treat my symptoms. When the tests came back, there was no sign of cancer.

Browsing in the book store one afternoon, I came across a new book on candida and yeast infections. This book talked about candida and how it could be treated with Nystatin. I was elated! Finally, I thought, I had the answer to my problems. All it was going to take was a little Nystatin and I was going to get well. I called my new doctor who wrote me a prescription.

But, I found that even ten years later, I was not cured.

In fact, all I really had to do was go off my very limited diet and eat a little sweets, sugar or ice cream and I would develop a rip-roaring candida infection, often accompanied by a staph infection. During this time, I also discovered homeopathy. As my recovery was painfully slow and uneven, Jai suggested that I consider homeopathy treatment.

So I was off to see a homeopathist. I was very intrigued by this man. He used some sort of machine to measure information from the acupuncture points on my finger and toes. He could tell which organs and meridians were not functioning properly and could identify the culprits: bacteria, viruses, fungus, etc., and make remedies to eliminate the offenders from the subtle bodies. It seemed pretty far out. But I was really suffering, I would try anything. After my initial skepticism was put aside, I found that I experienced dramatic relief from this treatment. He was able to eliminate the constant food poisoning and eventually the systemic staph infections that so drained my energy. He also identified and cleaned out many viruses from my system. Looking back, probably the most profound change in my health came from healing the blood staph. It had been responsible for constant kidney, bladder, and other infections I experienced. My energy and emotional well being increased tremendously when it was finally gone.

Although I was still living in Alaska, I was now separated from my husband and in the process of selling my real estate company. By now, I was too sick to work or do much of anything except lie in bed. I was tormented by a constant fatigue. I only had so much energy available. If I pushed myself too hard, I could not get out of bed. Also, I was experiencing a phenomenon where my adrenals would "blow out". I don't know how else to explain it. I could feel electrical energy go through my right kidney and my right adrenal would blow. When this happened, I would be flat on my back for weeks at a time. When the hair analysis came back, it indicated that I had no salt in my body. Later I was to learn this has something to do with adrenal exhaustion.

There was little communication between my husband and me during the two years we were separated. He refused to cooperate with my lawyer and ignored most of the requests and attempts at communication. I know that this was a very painful and difficult time for him as well. I was concerned about the boys. The older two boys were enrolled in a Catholic Boys High School in Colorado. They seemed to be happy there.

I was worried about the youngest. He was still in Jr. High when we separated. I was somewhat relieved when he chose to live with his father. I was so sick, I was afraid I could not handle the responsibility of taking care of him. Looking back, I have often felt this was a big mistake. Still in denial about his alcoholism, his father did a lot of drinking during this time. I felt this had tremendous psychological impact on Tim.

Tim's grades started to slip. He seemed confused and needed help. His father did not believe in anything like that. Just as soon as he was out of Jr. High, he was sent out to Colorado with his brothers. His personality changed. He started doing strange things. I was very concerned. I threatened to take him out of school. He pleaded with me not to embarrass him. So I made the choice that I have often regretted, and let him stay.

I went on a two week holistic retreat to Maui, sponsored by Jai Inder, and came back somewhat better. I was struck by the beauty there. I loved the warm sunlight and ocean. It was so peaceful and relaxing. This was just what I needed. I needed to live in a nurturing environment. During the retreat we learned skills for emotional and psychological release as well as nutrition and diet. We ate specially prepared organic food. Upon my return, I decided to move to Maui.

THE MOVE TO MAUI

It took several months to sell the furniture and personal possessions in the house. The whole idea of leaving was emotionally very upsetting. This was my life. I had saved everything. We lived in a large house in the woods on 2 1/2 acres for many years. In the spring, the moose wandered down from the mountains. Several calves had been born just outside our living room windows. I had built that house. The children had grown up and gone to school there. The thought of leaving was overwhelming. I realized that I had lived in Alaska for almost 25 years. If I were to ever leave it would be now. I was tired and sick. My marriage was over. My business was gone. The dark cold winters were very depressing to me. I was tired of dealing with the elements, including the ice and snow. Maui was calling me.

Methodically, I worked my way through the house, going through old boxes and mementos. I would have a garage sale every weekend, and go through a different room during the week. The process seemed to take forever. I found drawings and pictures the boys had done in nursery school. Everything was there. It was hard to dispose of things. I had to keep going. There would be little left for storage. The cost of shipping things to Maui was tremendous. I cried a lot.

Finally, the furniture was sold. The fur coats were put into storage. The business suits and cocktail dresses were sent off to the Salvation Army. The "for sale" sign was placed upon the house. I was starting a new chapter in my life. I did not know what was ahead for me. I just knew that I needed rest, lots of it.

The day finally came when I arrived in Maui. Let me say that I have traveled all over the world, and have yet to find a place on the planet that is more peaceful and rejuvenating to me. My soul truly feels at home on Maui. Many ancient traditions and legends tell us that Maui is one of the few land masses on the surface of earth remaining from ancient Lemuria. It feels that way to me. I have relived many ancient memories from that time in the history of the earth, including the grief of its destruction. Hawaiian legends say that it will rise again around the year 2000. Perhaps that is true. I don't know.

The island of Maui is in the shape of a woman's head and bust. I have always felt that this is the great mother goddess. She has left a reminder for all of us to see. She may be gone, and the virtues of love and caring that were associated with the great goddess civilization from the earliest days of earth may be forgotten, but she will return. Much of the lost science and knowledge from those times is being slowly retrieved. This includes the information involved with quantum physics, and vibrational healing. She still calls her people home to be healed.

Once in Maui, I immediately started to focus on the work at hand: getting well. I realized by now that traditional medicine was not going to work for me. I would waste away and slowly die if I were to wait for a cure from traditional means. No, something told me that if I was going to survive this ordeal, I was going to have to heal myself. I did not have the slightest clue as to how that would happen, but I trusted that there was some ancient force that would guide me. Perhaps it was the wisdom of the goddess herself, and I had to move there in order to be able to hear her voice. Perhaps it was my own ancient memory and wisdom that I was uncovering: knowledge that was being fed to me through my unconscious mind. Looking back now, I realize that I was guided forward step by step. I never could see beyond the present step, but that one was clearly provided for me. I just had to recognize the step and trust it.

Actually, there were two steps at hand. One was to focus on the physical body and the second was to release the emotional body. They both seemed important at the time.

EXPERIENCING PAST LIFE MEMORIES

The first thing I did was to contact some of the people I had met during the retreat. I had met a wonderful couple who were psychologists. So I looked them up and started working on myself. I did personal work and group work. I needed to work out many things in my life. I had a lot of anger with men. I spent years trying to understand and forgive my father. I had a lot of anger at my husband. I had a lot of anger at myself. I had always repressed my feelings, as it was not safe for me to express them. It was important to get in touch with my feelings. I did not know how it was going to happen, but I wanted to have feelings. I was to learn over time that these patterns were etched very deep in my soul. It was not simply a matter of working through my anger at my father in this life. My father had been my repressor in many lifetimes. I have traced this pattern back through the history of the earth and even lifetimes on other planets. This pattern has to do with the repression of the female energy on earth under the controlling philosophy of the patriarchy. It is ancient history that is tied in with the two polarized forces of positive and negative that keep our universe in balance.

This work was very important in my healing process. But I found that, initially, it had very little impact on my physical well being. In fact, there were many times when the releasing of anger and grief was overwhelming and added to the exhaustion and fatigue that I was already experiencing.

It was during this time that I began to experience a phenomenon in which past life memories would just "dump" into my consciousness. I remember the first time that it happened. I was sitting in a group. I don't remember what we were working on but all of a sudden, I was reliving being in England at the time of Henry VIII. I was being executed; my head was about to be chopped off. There were people there who had come to eat lunch, and I was the entertainment for the day. I was confused, embarrassed, and angry. I felt all the emotions of this very proud and confused woman.

This was very strange to me and I did not really understand what was happening. I later found that these lifetime experiences would just "dump in" and I did not have a lot of control over them. At a certain point in my life, my emotional body opened up and these memories began releasing. I found that the "real" world would stop and I would be trapped in the memories until I could release them and the emotions. So I began to investigate the different types of therapies that would facilitate me in releasing these past life memories. In the beginning, I worked with some people on Maui who did a process called "clear light therapy". They were clairvoyant and used crystals to lift energies from the subtle bodies. They would tell the stories they saw in the chakras as this energy was being lifted. Although it seemed to work, this was a very slow process. While reliving an ancient memory, I might be paralyzed in grief on the floor for eight hours at a time. I was remembering the destruction of Atlantis and Lemuria. I had a lot of grief about these times. I cried a lot.

This process continued during the time I lived in Maui. I had no control over how fast the memories came through. I never knew when the next one was coming. However, I learned to recognize the symptoms my physical body experienced when a lifetime memory dumped in and needed to be released. I called this process "being catalyzed".

I looked for quicker and easier ways to release this energy. I wanted to release the memories without experiencing all the emotions. I tried re-birthing and found that it was very time consuming. However, the breathing was a really good way to release stuck energy. It was an excellent tool to have. There were times when rebirthing was the most appropriate technique to use. I tried acupuncture and found that it also worked. Often, I would experience the memories as they were released during an acupuncture treatment. I worked with that for a time. It was another valuable tool.

Something needs to be said here about my experience with drugs. As I mentioned earlier, I was raised very traditionally. I was never exposed to drugs in any way. However, when I got to Maui, I found that most of the "spiritual" seekers there used drugs. This included most of the therapists and psychologists. The drugs of choice at that time included marijuana, LSD, and Ecstasy. Recently, South American plants known as Ayahuaska and Syrian Rue have increased in popularity. Everybody used them. I resisted. I was afraid of drugs. I had read about horrible things that happened to people on drugs.

My closest friend kept inviting me to have the experience with her. I resisted for a long time. Finally, I agreed to have the experience with the drug known as Ecstasy only after being assured by my psychologists that it was a legal substance. I was also told that many miraculous healings had taken place with the substance. Reluctantly, I finally agreed to try it. I was pretty terrified of what might happen to me. Would I lose control of my feelings and emotions? Perhaps I would act crazy and weird. Would I have a "bad trip"? Could it affect my brain and thinking process?

In all fairness, I have to say that it truly was an amazing experience. I remember sitting in the swing on the porch of my friend's house when my heart chakra opened up and lifetimes of memories poured out. One by one, I recalled the details of lifetimes when I had been imprisoned, executed, burned at the stake, and beheaded. This went on for hours. Finally, they stopped. I was greatly relieved. Then I forgave everyone, including my father, as I had seen that he had been my imprisoner and executor in many lifetimes. What an experience! It was truly healing. I was totally exhausted. A ton of bricks had been lifted off my emotional body. The truly amazing fact was that my father, who had been an invalid for 15 years, died the next day! He was waiting for me to forgive him. I had not been able to say the words until now.

I began working with a small group of friends releasing past life memories with Ecstasy. We met once every two months for a year or so. I was taught to pray over the substance and call in the light, then set the intention to release a certain chakra. The healings were often profound. I was impressed. I was also concerned about getting addicted to the substance, and took smaller and smaller doses of the drug. Over time, I found that I did not have to take any drug, that I could "see" and release the information simply by being with others who had taken the drug. Eventually, I reached a place when there were no more releases on the drug. I stopped. At some point during that time, the drug Ecstasy was classified as an "illegal" substance. So much for drugs. I cannot emphasize the point enough – taking drugs for any reason is a big mistake. The negatives far outweigh the positives. I have made the decision: no more drugs of any kind. For me personally, this includes prescription drugs as well.

SHAMANISTIC HEALING

There seems to be a lot of interest today in this type of healing. It has come to be known as Shamanistic healing although I seriously doubt that the "pure" practice of this art involves drugs. Loosely defined, I would describe it as the use of drugs or hallucinogenic substances to take journeys into other dimensions and release and heal memories of the past. I personally think that the dangers involved are much greater than the healings gained. The real danger of drugs lies in that fact that they can take you into dimensions and feelings that are almost impossible to experience without them. Feeling a oneness with the universe and the love that exists can be very alluring.

The other side is more subtle and hidden. This is the side that involves dark forces and energies that exist on other planes and dimensions.

Most of the people that I have personally met who lead these journeys are really substance abusers. They do not realize that the dark forces that they meet on the journeys are attached to the drugs and chemicals in their bodies. Many people become "possessed" by dark energies or entities as a result of these "trips". I have also met people who have blown their psychic shield on drugs. This is serious business as it affects your mental balance. Drugs are very dangerous things to do. I do not recommend this type of healing to anyone.

I have learned a lot about drugs in my work. I do not do drugs anymore, for any reason. Nor do I work with, or hang out with people who do them. There are three reasons for this. One is that drugs are illegal substances. The current laws involving drugs give law enforcement agencies tremendous power. Even occasional usage of drugs could cost you your auto, home, boat, or other property. You need to ask yourself, "Is this worth the risk?" The second reason is that drugs are addictive. Anyone using drugs for any reason runs the risk of addiction. And the third reason is that they may be contaminated by lethal herbicides and toxic solvents that could lead to AIDS, CFIDS or other immune dysfunction disease.

Research with the "SE5" (special sound equipment) indicates that drugs and chemicals of all kinds, once ingested into the body, will leave behind residues that build up in the cells and tissues of the body. This white, granular substance will crystallize and get very hard. It will clog the small blood vessels, arteries and the glands that secrete hormones. The residue will also end up in the fat and fatty tissues of the body, including the brain. As this substance builds up in the body, it will create holes in the aura or energy field around the body.

The aura is our only protection from astral energies and beings living on other planes. These holes allow astral energies to come right in and make themselves at home in our bodies. This is how people get possessed. Certain "dark force" groups resonate with the different chemicals in the drugs. As long as those chemicals are in the body, these beings will be around and able to influence situations in your life. Also, I am finding that certain viruses seem to grow off the drugs. So if you are tempted to use drugs, read this book first. It may save you a lot of grief and confusion.

USING HYPNOSIS TO CLEAR PAST LIFE TRAUMAS

I have learned that hypnosis can produce similar results without the dangers involved with drugs. I became certified in hypnosis and have developed a program using regression hypnosis that will quickly clear traumatic lifetime memories, release controlling entities and spirit forms, and clear karmic situations. It is faster and more effective than any drug, without the dangers. Although past life regression therapy is becoming very acceptable today, it seems important to state that very few therapists knew anything about it ten years ago. I was often ridiculed and scolded for "exploring" past lives when I had many things to work out in this life. The fact that I had no control over what was happening seemed of little consequence. Five years later, these same therapists would be flying off to California to take classes and seminars from Stan Groff and raving about the process. Today, I am very thankful that others have come to know the value of hypnosis as a healing tool.

I find that many people have misconceived ideas about hypnosis and how it will affect them. We have all seen the nightclub acts where people do weird things on stage. Many people feel that they will end up doing something stupid, or go away somewhere and not be aware of what happens to them. First let me say, that you will not do anything that does not feel appropriate, and you will re-member everything that goes on during the session. I provide audio tapes of the session if the client feels good about recording what happens during a session. Often it is good to go home and re-listen to the experience. New insight can be gained this way.

Think of hypnosis as a guided visualization or medita-tion that allows you to get very relaxed so that you can get in touch with information buried in your unconscious mind. It is this unconscious information that tends to influence the experiences and decisions you have every day. Hypnosis is an excellent way to clean out your closet, or basement. First you have to make up your mind to do something about cleaning it up. Then you need to go into the basement and begin to look at all the junk that has been stored there over lifetimes. Once you have taken inventory, you may begin to realize that there is much stored there that you have outgrown, or that is holding you back in certain patterns or ways of being. With hypnosis, you can identify each pattern, understand where it has come from and how it is affecting your life today, then decide if it is in your best interest to hold on to this old pattern. Perhaps you would like to throw it out and make room for a new experience.

Old repressed emotions can be released easily and quickly. I find that so many people hang on to huge emotional blocks out of fear of facing and dealing with the emotions. Sometimes these experiences are very traumatic and painful. Believe me, one good cry can create miracles in your life. Once on the other side, you will look back and wonder why you resisted for so long.

Like any tool, it can and has been misused throughout the ages. It is important that you find a therapist that you feel good about. Take your time to shop around. Make sure that the therapist you chose does not take drugs or abuses other substances. Not all therapists have their act together. Take some time to investigate and chose the right one.

I spent the first four years in Maui crying and releasing grief. Sometimes my grief felt like a bottomless pit. When would this ever stop? There were always more memories and more grief. I felt I was a personification of the feminine spirit that was continuously repressed, imprisoned, and victimized by negative forces that control the world. How did this all start? I wanted to know why it happened as it did.

40

Somewhere along the line, I began to realize that there was a story that could be put together from these memories. For the most part, they seemed to be moving backwards through time. I began to record the information. During the fifteen years that I have been doing this work, I have relived much of my history with the planet earth. It is a very ancient history. I have remembered much about the things that have happened here. Perhaps, someday, I will tell this story.

TAKING CARE OF THE PHYSICAL BODY

I also educated myself about alternative or holistic medicine. I searched out practitioners who could help me keep my physical body in check. This included energy work, supplements, herbs, and homeopathy. I worked with naturopathic medicine, acupuncture, nutritionists, and chiropractors. I saw and experienced many types of practitioners. I wanted to personally experience all types of healing therapies so that I could determine which were the most effective for me.

On several occasions, I was asked if I had ever been addicted to drugs. I was surprised and replied "no". (My limited experience with drugs was to come later.) I was told that conditions existed in my body that were similar to those experienced by a drug addict. I had the body of a habitual drug user! How could that be? I was told at one point that I had "pin point pupils"—that my pupils did not dilate properly. This did not mean anything to me until much later in my research. I also had indications of cancer in my subtle bodies show up continuously. I was regularly given remedies for cancer. Still nothing showed up on the blood tests.

I had lots of massage and body work. I swam every day. I loved walking on the beach and smelling the ocean. I watched my diet very carefully, and I got lots and lots of rest. I lived on a very restricted diet of steamed vegetables and small amounts of protein. I found that as long as I stayed on this simple diet, my body functioned fairly well. However, the minute I added milk products, or sweets to my diet, I would develop a candida infection or a staph infection. Popcorn was the only treat that my body would allow. If I followed this routine very carefully, my symptoms would not get worse, but I did not get any better either.

Under threat of constant bladder and kidney infections, my research into homeopathic medicine led me to a therapist who used an Intero machine to map the acupuncture points of my body and create remedies with a much more sophisticated computer than in my experience in Alaska. Traditional antibiotics would activate the candida, so I used homeopathy. It was very effective for me. I knew intuitively that if I could afford one of these machines, I would be able to heal myself. However, the price tag of $25,000 was more than I could afford. So I put the thought into the back of my mind.

By 1988, my health was somewhat stabilized. The lifetime memories had slowed down considerably, allowing me three to four weeks between "dumps". I had learned how to keep my body functioning at a fairly stable level. I had learned to listen to my body for signs and indications of just how far I could go before I risked a system blowout. I had a whole regimen of vitamins, herbs and remedies I ingested every day. But more importantly, I knew exactly what to do if this happened, or that happened. Armed with my new level of body function, I felt it was time for the next step.

Money became a concern. I had not worked in almost 6 years. I was living on my real estate assets, converting property into cash by selling it. My cash resources were getting very depleted. I was easily spending $10,000 a year on my health. The financial cost to me to date, not including lost opportunities to make money, has easily been $500,000. This is the dollar figure I can put on living very conservatively for twelve years without income, including therapists, herbs, supplements and equipment.

I needed to think about a new career so that I would be prepared when the money ran out. So, I decided to move again, this time to California. I had always seen that my work would involve healing with color and sound, so I decided it was time to learn about technology.

I enrolled in Computer Arts Institute in San Francisco to learn about graphic arts and video computers. I also spent several years doing volunteer work at Viacom Community Access Television where I learned about video and television production.

I also met and began working with Brenda Bastys, a very remarkable lady who was a hypnotherapist and clairvoyant. She had developed the most amazing clearing techniques, and was possibly the most accurate psychic

43

that I had ever met. Thus began an association that lasted for over three years. During that time, I worked with her regularly at least once a week.

Brenda could read the past life information in the chakras and subtle bodies, and clear them at the same time. I began to tape all the sessions as there was so much information. She could retrieve the smallest details. Sometimes we worked in a hypnotic trance, but for the most part, she could see a lot more of the details than I could, so I let her read and clear the information. I was excited by the idea that I did not actually have to relive the experience. This was new for me, and it saved on my energy. I have boxes of audio tapes from her sessions. With persistence, there will be more books.

MY CALIFORNIA EXPERIENCE

In the beginning, my life was very much a continuation of Maui, balancing work with rest. I was living alone with little energy to make friends or do social activities. However, I was excited and delighted to have the energy to go to school at night and felt I was surely on my way to recovery. Time was to tell that I had gotten too optimistic about my recovery. By the spring of 1989, I was sick again. Really sick. In fact, I was worse than when I left Alaska for Maui.

Confident of my new health, I had let my diet slip. I was eating bread and sweets. I loved ice cream. I allowed myself to indulge in it. Occasionally, I had a glass of wine. I was drinking tap water. I had not spent the money to purchase a water purifier. I was not aware at the time just how important this was.

I was living in Novato, California near a military base. Once I became aware of the dangers from military bases, I began to analyze the water with my SE5. I became very alarmed at the type of toxic chemical residues in the water. This included Agent Orange and other herbicides as well as other toxic chemicals. At first, I was reluctant to believe that this was possible. It seemed unbelievable. I must have made a mistake. Where could this be coming from? I checked into the costs of having the water analyzed by a testing facility, and dismissed that thought as out of the question; I could not afford the fee. More than likely, tests would have come back negative, just like my blood tests. We are dealing with chemical residues here, residues of chemicals that are so subtle they may not be detected on the physical plane. However, these residues will accumulate and build up in the cells of the body. Eventually, they are able to cause disease and affect the physical body.

Once again, I was back spending big bucks on therapists. I was struggling with staph and strep infections. My energy was low. I was really depressed. For the first time in this process, I was beginning to give up. I was losing my desire to fight back. I was tired of holding on. Perhaps it was time to let go and admit that there was no cure for this disease. I was just going to die slowly. I was not sure that anybody cared. I would just waste away until I died. I hoped that the end would come soon as I was running out of money. This new bout of illness brought real concerns about how I was going to manage and live the rest of my life.

Then two very miraculous things happened. The phone rang one day. It was a friend from Maui, Dr. Irv Katz. A Ph.D. psychologist, Irv had been my hypnosis teacher. He was in town with his girlfriend and wanted to share some information with me. Could we meet at the Holiday Inn for lunch? Yes, most definitely. I was always happy to have visitors.

Ennula, his girlfriend, also suffered from CFIDS. Sometimes we shared information about therapies we had tried. She had recently bought an ozone machine and was pursuing that therapy. She had some success with chelation therapy and was anxious to share her experiences with me. Over lunch, they introduced me to a machine called the SE5. Based on scaler energy technology it was similar to the Intero machine that I had worked with in Maui. I was excited when I found that the price was $2,500. It would be a stretch, but I could afford one. I knew that with this device I would be able to research and discover what I needed to know to complete my healing. I renewed my hope that I might be cured. So I ordered a machine on the spot.

HTLV I & 2 VIRUSES

While I was anxiously awaiting the arrival of the SE5, I happened to read an article in the newspaper talking about an epidemic at Johns Hopkins University School of Medicine in Baltimore. Two cancer causing viruses, were threatening health-care workers at the hospital. Once confined to a Japanese island, the Caribbean, Africa & Southeast Italy, these viruses were rare ten years go, but were spreading throughout the U.S. since 1985.

Studies indicated that 1% of all patients admitted to Johns Hopkins' emergency room in 1988 tested positive for HTLV I & 2 infection (human T-lymphotropic viruses types 1 & 2). By comparison, 6% of the same population tested positive for AIDS virus infection. While the AIDS virus was concentrated among homosexual men and intravenous drug users, HTLV I & 2 infections were found in a broad cross-section of the patient population. An alarming number of HTLV I & 2 infections were found in elderly patients, who were not drug users. No one knew how these elderly people had contacted the virus. Recent San Francisco studies showed that 3% of women admitted at a local hospital for pelvic inflammatory disease were infected with HTLV I & 2.

The article went on to say that HTLV-1 is a very slow-acting virus that can infect people 20-30 years before causing disease. Then it may produce a type of cancer of the immune system, a neurological pain disorder, or another nerve disorder that is marked by destruction of the protective sheaths around the nerves. Research had yet to pinpoint a specific disease related to HTLV 2. An AIDS family virus, health care workers were in danger of contracting the virus from infected blood just as AIDS might be contracted.[1]

Something told me to cut this out. A voice inside said, "This is what you are looking for, this is the key to getting well." Today, as a result of my work, I am convinced that these viruses are directly connected with plutonium and other forms of radiation exposure and poison. I cannot prove it by traditional scientific means, but I feel that in time, the scientific community will get around to finding this out for themselves. Although my methods of research are non-traditional, they are effective and totally responsible for my recovery. I am sure it is only a matter of time before my findings are "proven" by the traditional scientific community.

The second miracle in my life was in the fall of 1989, when I met the man who is my life mate today. His name is Angelo, Italian for Angel, and he is truly just that. He brought new hope and courage into my life at a time when I needed it the most. He helped me through the critical months that lay ahead, when on several occasions I almost died. He has continued to support me in the face of much opposition, never losing faith in my knowledge and the truth of my work. With him I have found the love and the intimacy that I longed for with my mate. I love him and thank him.

PART 2

My Personal

Research

PART 2

MY PERSONAL RESEARCH

SE5 Biofield Spectrum Analyzer

The SE5 belongs to the field of energy medicine. This new science deals with the electrical or electromagnetic energy surrounding the physical body, known as the subtle bodies, or biofield.

Ancient philosophies of healing believed that dis-ease manifested in the physical body had its origins in the subtle bodies which were less dense in makeup than the physical. Health, they believed, depended upon the free flow of energy in the subtle bodies.

The principals of this science, although very ancient, were lost somewhere in history and are being remembered or rediscovered today. The electrical, or electromagnetic energy surrounding the physical body has many names, including life force, chi, scaler wave, and prana.

Recent advances have created technology allowing researchers to influence subtle electrical energies in the aura around the body. This technology analyzes and measures information in the subtle bodies, allowing imbalances to be released, thereby changing the energetic qualities of the physical body.

In recent years machines have been designed to identify and read electrical and electromagnetic energy. Machines include radionics, Interos, Orgone Accumulators, Psychotronic

Generators, Biofeedback machines, Nutritrons, Vitrons and Digitrons.

Invented by Willard Frank, the SE5 is a solid state electronic instrument designed to detect, quantify and transmit subtle energy signals, allowing for the balancing and restoring of harmonious wave form patterns in the aura. The SE5 does not act directly on the physical body, but works with the subatomic patterns or magnetic energy in the pre-physical state (biofield or aura). This instrument assists the operator in creating an electronic link with mind/body energies. Once the link is established, energies can be released that have a detrimental effect and then remaining energies balanced to enhance the overall well being and normalization of the physical body.[2]

It, like many similar devices, is considered experimental by the FDA, and no claims can be made for its effectiveness. My intention is to simply convey to you my personal experience and my research with this device. It has proven most accurate in my case. I owe my life to this device.

THE SEARCH FOR A VIRUS

I waited anxiously for my new machine to arrive. My physical condition worsened. I developed new symptoms. My body was not metabolizing fat. My cholesterol levels were very high. Something very intense was happening to my nervous system. I was experiencing a lot of bleeding with my periods. They were more like hemorrhages than periods. None of the usual herbs or supplements seemed to work. The stress showed on my face. I was aging rapidly.

I began to work with a nutritionist who was an expert with radionics and scaler technology. When the SE5 arrived, I ran to an appointment at his office and asked that he teach me how to work this device. In the process, would he please use the machine to see if he could identify what was happening to me? I showed him the newspaper article. Did I have these HTLV viruses in my system?

Several days later, he called back with the news. Yes, he had found indications of the presence of HTLV viruses in my system in really high amounts. He explained that these viruses are all a family of AIDS viruses. The viruses that were indicated in my case were HTLV 1 & 2. He knew of no treatment. I asked about the chances of clearing the viruses with the SE5. He responded saying that he had known people who had successfully eliminated viruses from their systems with the SE5, but it usually took a year or longer. I did not have a year. He suggested ozone treatments. He had clients who had reported success in controlling HTLV viruses with ozone treatments. I told him I would think about it and let him know my decision.

I did not like the idea of putting ozone into my body. Something bothered me about it. I called him the next day and said that I wanted to try working with the SE5 first. Something told me that it would work. We made an appointment to get together. He showed me how the machine worked and how to go about broadcasting to eliminate the specific viruses from my system. I thanked him and set about my own personal research with the SE5.

To our amazement, the viruses did not take the usual year that he expected, but were gone from my system in 3-4 days. He was truly amazed! Why was this happening? I was excited. Perhaps it was all the releasing work that I had done over the years. Perhaps by clearing my subtle bodies, I had released the density of the physical body. I did not carry around the density, the vibrational weight that most people carried.

This was the only explanation that we could find that made any sense. All the release work I had done to the present time was preparing me for the moment. Since the SE5 works with the operator's energy, the clearer the operator, the higher the vibrational frequency of the operator, the faster the machine will clear negative influences. Eventually, I did not need the device at all. Today, I only use it to identify specific frequencies of offending substances. Once identified, I can clear these influences faster than the SE5 simply by focusing my attention to clear them.

Keep in mind that the SE5 works by accessing and identifying information from the subtle bodies. It can detect the vibrational presence of certain energies. It cannot tell you whether these energies are active or inactive in the physical body. In my research, it was enough for me to identify the presence of a substance. I was not concerned with the fact of whether it was physically active in the body. I was very clear to point out that I did not do diagnosis of this type. That is the function of blood tests. When I talk about finding the presence of a virus or bacteria, I am talking about its vibration being present in the subtle energy field. Once located, it can be eliminated, whether it is active or not.

I started identifying viruses in my subtle bodies and systematically went about eliminating them. There were lots of different viruses, including Epstein Barr, herpes, mononucleosis, hepatitis, coxsackie, cytomeglovato and others. The list was very long. Next, I started in on the bacteria, eliminating staph, strep and other bacteria. There were many present including mycobacteria, spirochete, and anaerobic. Then on to funguses and parasites. Methodically, I went through the SE5 manual, listing and eliminating organisms in my subtle bodies. Within several weeks, I was starting to feel alive again. My hope and excitement returned with my new found energy. Perhaps my inner guidance was right again. I was going to cure myself of this disease!

I bought all the books I could find on viruses and theories involved in AIDS and Chronic Fatigue Syndrome.

There was not much on Chronic Fatigue Syndrome which helped my research, but there were lots of books offering theories and information on viruses. I started reading.

As I researched these viruses. I found that the HTLV 1 & 2 viruses, obscure ten to twelve years ago, could attack the nervous system and eventually cause a rare form of leukemia. In fact, there were six viruses in the HTLV family, HTLV 3 and HIV were the same virus. In my research, trying to locate and identify a virus, or family of viruses, that might be the cause of CFIDS, I was convinced that the HTLV viruses were the most likely candidates.

You can imagine my disappointment when several months later, the viruses and funguses I had so carefully eliminated from my body started growing back again. I spent several years working with different theories about why this was happening. Since HTLV viruses were retroviruses, they tended to mutate very quickly. I felt that somehow I was missing some of the mutations and this is why the viruses were growing back.

It was during this time, that my health took a turn for the worse and I almost died. My periods had become very heavy, they were more like hemorrhages than periods. One morning I awoke to find myself in a huge pool of blood. There was blood all over the bed, all over me. I was weak and dizzy. I had left my body and was floating around the room. The phone rang. I had great difficulty getting to it. Finally, with a great deal of effort, I managed to pick it up and say "hello". Angelo, my boyfriend, was on the other end. He asked, "What was happening with me." I was not too coherent, but murmured something about blood everywhere.

Alarmed, he wanted to come over and take me to the hospital. I did not want to go to the hospital. I had no insurance, I could not afford it. Besides, I was afraid that they would give me a blood transfusion. I might get AIDS. That would be the last straw. I did not want to have anything to do with doctors or hospitals. I had no faith in either one.

Besides, I was tired of living. I was tired of the fight to live. I just wanted to leave and go back to that beautiful place where I had been before. There was no love here. No one cared. I could not get well. I just wanted to die. He was pretty desperate. I was not making any sense to him, but I was making perfect sense to me. I was out of my body and ready to go. He threatened to call an ambulance as he was at least an hour and a half's drive from my place.

I hung up and floated around the room some more. I became concerned about him calling an ambulance. I definitely could not afford that!

Remembering that I had died once before and was not allowed to stay in "heaven", I became more rational. Perhaps that would happen again. If the ambulance took me to the hospital, I could end up with a blood transfusion, or worse, they might operate on me.

I did not like that thought. I made a decision that I had better do something about the bleeding. I called a woman herbalist. I asked what herbs I needed to take to stop the bleeding. She recommended several. I wrote them down. Very slowly and with a lot of effort, I began to think about getting to the health food store which was not too far away. With great effort, I was able to dress. I was very dizzy and weak so I walked very slowly. Eventually, I got into my car and drove to pick up the herbs.

Once home again, I rested for a while, then began brewing the herbal tea using these blood clotting herbs. I drank some tea and went back to bed. I tried to find a place where there was no blood. I was too tired to change the bed. I passed out. Periodically, I would wake up and drink tea. This went on for most of the day. That afternoon, Angelo arrived, very concerned about what he might find.

I was definitely weak, but the bleeding had slowed down. The tea was working. I drank as much as I could for another day. By the end of the second day, the bleeding had stopped. I had lost a lot of blood, however, and was very weak. I was having trouble getting back into my body. It was a very strange experience to find that most of me was outside of my body and could not find a way back in. I found that everything I did was a great effort. It felt like I was dragging my body along everywhere. So strange. I remained this way until I went to an acupuncturist who could tell this was happening by reading the pulses. She stimulated the point at the top of my head to let me back into my body. Boy, what a relief that was!

Making the decision to stay around did nothing for

my mental state. I was at my wit's end. I truly felt that I was developing leukemia at this time in my life. Something needed to happen quickly. I was running out of time. I increased the time I spent in research. I worked like I was possessed. I worked night and day with little rest.

I was working on my son, Tim, as well. During this same time, he had experienced a physical and emotional breakdown and had to be taken out of school. He was back in Alaska with his father undergoing major tests.

I found almost identical conditions in his system to mine, including the HTLV viruses. I worked night and day to clean his system out. Perhaps, I could buy him some time.

All this happened in September of 1990. Several months later, I had an experience that, to this day, I feel has to be one of the most bizarre and terrifying experiences that anyone could undergo.

VISIT BY EXTRATERRESTRIALS

It was early Sunday morning after Thanksgiving. I awoke in the early hours of the day totally paralyzed. At first I thought I was dreaming. I decided, no, I was awake. I was talking to myself. I was aware of being in my bed and the things in the bedroom. However, I could not move any part of me except my eyes. I was filled with a strange terror I had never experienced before, but I was still able to think. I thought, "This is strange, what is happening here?" I turned my eyes to the right side of the bed, and my heart skipped a few beats. There appeared to be a strange human-like creature with large slanted almond black eyes. This creature was communicating with me telepathically, threatening my life. Basically, it told me to stop what I was doing, or I would not live much longer. It took me a while to comprehend this; I was in total shock. Finally, I got really angry. I found myself communicating telepathically with him stating, "What could you do to me that you have not already done? How dare you?" (Later, I was to ponder what I meant by these words.) Just then I heard a voice in my head say, "You are in control here, use your will."

I started repeating to myself: "I am in control, this being cannot harm me." I called in the light of Jesus Christ. Suddenly the being disappeared. It was gone. Vanished. I was no longer paralyzed, I could move.

Believe me, I was confused and in shock. What was this? How could this be? I called Angelo. I paced around the room. Part of me just wanted to flee. What if this thing came back? Believe me, this was more terrorizing than all of the pain and sickness I had experienced to date. Was I hallucinating? Definitely not. I was awake the whole time.

After I calmed down and had a chance to think, I realized that I had seen a face like this on the cover of a book that someone had given to me years ago. It was in my book case. I had never taken the time to read the book. I walked into the living room and began looking for the book. There it was. I pulled it out to look at the cover. The word **Communion**[3] stared at me along with this strange face. Yes. These two beings were very similar

60

looking. Perhaps it was time to read this book. I sat down right there and began. The thought of beings coming into my house at will was very frightening. Would they come back?

As I retraced my experience in my mind, I realized that these beings did not walk down my hallway into my bedroom. Suddenly they were there, then they were gone. I recalled some of my work with past life memories of extraterrestrial groups. I remembered that they often used holographic technology to project into spaces. This had to be a holographic projection, but where did it come from? Who is behind this? Was I to believe that some extraterrestrial beings, from the Zeta Reticula, were just in my bedroom, threatening my life? Why were they concerned about my research into viruses and Chronic Fatigue Syndrome? I felt really confused and afraid. What if they came back? Had I been abducted and experimented with like the experiences in **Communion**? If so, what had they done to me? I had a lot of questions.

I lived with the curtains closed for several weeks. I was hiding out. I was terrified that these beings would return. Although I realized that closing the curtains would not keep them out, somehow I felt more secure. Looking back, I realize I was not acting too rational at the time. However, this was not a rational experience.

My anxiety drove me to attempt to share this experience with others. I made the mistake of telling my oldest son about the experience. He was convinced that someone should come and get me with a straight jacket. That increased my anxiety level. No one wanted to believe me, again.

Thank God, Angelo believed me. He was the first person I called immediately following the experience. He felt my terror. He knew it was real. After a while, I stopped needing to talk about the experience.

Shortly after their visit, I started experiencing very severe symptoms. Something incredible was happening to my nervous system. I don't know how to explain it, but it felt that someone had increased the voltage running through my nervous system. The voltage was somehow turned up so high that it was shorting out my system. It felt like I had stuck my finger into a high voltage socket. Without warning, I would have these attacks. They were so intense, I knew I was going to die for sure.

When I looked in the mirror, I found that I had aged 20 years in two weeks. What could they have done to me that produced this effect? I had no idea, but I was going to find out. I started reading UFO information about abductions. There were several books with valuable information on the market. I was surprised at the number of people who reported encounters with ETs, including abductions.

One day, as I was poring over a book, hoping for a clue to my predicament, something popped out of the page. The passage stated that one of the cruelest things that these beings will do is to implant victims with plutonium crystals in their brain, behind the pineal gland. This had the effect of keeping them in their body and was very detrimental to their overall well being.[4] Detrimental all right! Plutonium would kill most humans by causing leukemia or cancer.

Could that be possible? Could I have plutonium crystals implanted in my brain? Why would anyone do such a thing? Could that be the explanation for this sudden and painful experience with my nervous system? I got out my SE5 and began searching for plutonium crystals. To my astonishment, I found plutonium crystals in my brain and in the rectum. It was not an easy task, but eventually, I was able to break them down and eliminate them from my body. I experienced immediate relief from these symptoms. My nervous system was nowhere near normal, but the painful sensation of being "fried" left. I was never to experience it again.

Since my experience in 1990, there have been many books and television shows with information from others who have reported very similar experiences. A Roper Survey conducted in 1992 involving 6000 adult Americans, suggested that hundreds of thousands, if not millions of American men, women and children may have experienced UFO abductions, or abduction related phenomena. This survey was part of a report sent to mental health professionals and was a joint effort by a Professor of Psychiatry at Harvard Medical School, a Professor of Sociology at Eastern Michigan University, and an Associate Professor of History at Temple University, a psychiatric therapist in Springfield, Missouri, and a researcher from New York City.[5]

Since this visit, I have gathered much information from clients to add to my own personal experience. The results of my research have enabled me to assist others who do not wish to be abducted. There seem to be many factors involved, including plutonium. Since that time, I have helped many people who have come to me with memories of being abducted or visited by extraterrestrial groups.

I don't pretend to have all the answers, but I have learned a great deal about this phenomenon. There seem to be certain things that tie this experience in with CFIDS and AIDS. Most clients seem to have one or more of the following in common: 1) high levels of radiation in their bodies; this includes plutonium and strontium 90, 2) the presence of toxic solvents, including toxic red water and/or other types of solvents, 3) a history of drug usage, 4) report experience happening after use of drugs or alcohol, 5) presence of high levels of HTLV viruses in abductions associated with Zeta Reticuli, 6) presence of AIDS virus in abductions associated with ETs known as Dracos, 7) some past genetic or ancestrial connection to abductors.

Information that I have gained concerning the extraterrestrials from the Zeta Reticuli who are most commonly associated with abductions includes the fact that they are from planets that have been destroyed by nuclear holocaust. They have high levels of radiation and viruses in their bodies as a result of this occurrence. Supposedly, they are attempting to create a hybrid race between humans and Zetas in order to fortify the breakdown of their DNA that they are experiencing because of radiation levels.

Many organs of their bodies are already atrophied,

including the digestive and sexual. I don't want to get into this in detail here, but I would like to point out the connection to high levels of radiation and the HTLV viruses, as this situation is usually also present in the people they choose to abduct. In certain instances, this environment may be artificially induced by the implantation of plutonium and viruses within the humans in an attempt to create an environment which is more conducive to the survival of the fetus.

For the most part, I feel that most abductees already have the desirable radiated environment in their physical bodies that make them likely targets. I do know that people who have high levels of radiation and viruses in their body are more likely to be abductees. This would indicate that somewhere along the line, they have experienced exposure to plutonium or other forms of radiation that would produce the virus environment in their bodies. Clearly, this means that they have been exposed to high levels of plutonium somewhere in their genetic lineage, including this lifetime, or past incarnations including lifetimes of ancestors.

What could be the source of such exposure? How could it be possible that so many people could be exposed to amounts of radiation high enough to cause the viruses that could eventually produce leukemia and other forms of radiation cancer?

I believe there are several possible scenarios that could explain this situation. I will present them for your consideration. The first one involves exposure to contaminated drugs. As I mentioned earlier, I am finding subtle energy indications that drugs may be contaminated with lethal substances including plutonium, nerve gas chemicals/pesticides and other solvents. Some prescription drugs that I have tested are contaminated with residues of toxic chemicals as well .

The second scenario involves recent information from the Department of Energy indicating that the U.S. government, after World War II between 1948 and 1952, deliberately dropped radioactive material from planes or released it on the ground in over a dozen experiments. Known test sites include Tennessee, Utah, New Mexico, Oregon and Washington state. In many of these tests, radiation spread beyond the planned boundaries of test. In the fall of 1949, the Army dropped cluster bombs containing radiation particles reaching 1500 curies from a plane flying at 15,000 feet. That level of radiation could cause death to those exposed at extremely close range in about an hour.[6]

Just suppose that the millions of people suffering from CFIDS were exposed to doses of radiation that were not lethal, but were strong enough to cause symptoms of leukemia to appear 20-30 years after initial exposure. That might account for the high numbers involved here. One must also look at the possibility that CFIDS victims have accumulated small doses of radiation from contaminated water and soil as a result of these tests. Foods grown in soil contaminated by radioactive fallout, as well as products from contaminated animals, could cause serious health problems many years later. Residues of these toxic substances accumulate in the tissues and build up gradually. Over the years, CFIDS victims may have accumulated enough radiation to show symptoms of radiation poisoning, developing a variety of viruses which could lead to serious disease, including CFIDS, cancer, or leukemia.

The third possibility is that millions of people have been exposed to radiation from nuclear waste dump sites that have resulted in the contamination of water and food supplies.

We also need to consider the possibility that the government's secret nuclear program that involved injecting unsuspecting Americans with doses of radiation is a lot more massive than indicated in recent disclosures. Personally, I think there is much more to come to light in this area.

Finally, we need to look at the possibility that there is some genetic influence involved from past incarnations where there was some experience with radiation. Many times, during hypnosis, clients will remember lifetimes on the very planets the Zetas are from. Therefore, there seems to be some genetic connection with the Zetas that makes them candidates for selection as breeders. Most all of my CFIDS clients will remember experiences where they have died in nuclear or atomic disasters on this planet or in other worlds. Radiation contamination from these lifetimes seems to have a very real influence on the conditions experienced in their body today.

I feel that the Zetas are drawn here today because of the high radiation levels on our planet. In a sense, they are the natural inheritors of this planet if things keep going in the same direction they have been going. We will begin to look more and more like the Zetas as we, as a species, begin to experience the breakdown of our genes and genetic material due to radiation. Perhaps the Zetas have plans to move in just as soon as the radiation levels are high enough. Suppose the hybrid race they are creating is a front-runner, or advance team, which will act as liaisons.

Since the Zetas cannot survive in oxygenated environments, they are creating a race that will be able to do that, a transition team, so to speak. I know all of this is very frightening to most people. However, denial never solved anything. The truth is that millions of Americans are having very similar experiences that involve these beings. Whether it is a third dimensional reality, or a reality caused by the plutonium and radiation in the brains of the ones having the experiences, I do not know for sure. I can only speak to my own experience. It was very real, and involved some form of holographic projection. That is all I know for sure.

It is my experience that most abductions can be stopped. Inevitably, there seems to be a karmic connection from the past. I have helped many others to find and release this connection, thereby stopping the experience of abduction. It is important, however, to clear the physical body of radiation and implants as well.

Also, as a word of warning, I do not suggest that anyone who reads this book is qualified to release victims from abduction experiences. This warning most definitely applies to other therapists in the field. This can prove to be a very dangerous situation. It is important that you do a lot of clearing on yourself first. Otherwise, the abducting ETs may decide to abduct you as well. NO ONE IS IMMUNE FROM ABDUCTIONS.

MY WORK WITH OTHERS

In July, 1991, I returned to Maui for an extended visit. In light of all that had happened the previous fall, Angelo was having some serious doubts about a long term association with me. This was pretty way out stuff. My experiences and research methods were testing him to the limits. I decided that I really could not stay in Marin as there were too many memories here. Many of them were of pain and suffering and defeat. Others were of triumph and joy. There was much love and joy in our relationship, and I would miss it too much. I could not stand to be here. So, once again, I mustered up all the strength I could manage and began packing for Maui. I could not stay in California.

Maui was a disappointment too. I was upset at the changes that I found upon my return. The biggest upset was the discovery that drugs were everywhere. Many of my friends were doing drugs all the time. That bothered me a lot. I had nobody to hang out with. The other disappointment was the impact that the economic recession had on everyone and everything. Maui did not seem to hold the same magic for me. I missed Angelo, too.

I spent a lot of time by myself. I did not socialize

much. I would wake early in the morning for a long walk along the beach, have a quick breakfast and start my day. I was totally involved in my work.

Once there, I started to do research with others who had CFIDS, spending hours identifying viruses, funguses, and bacteria, then spending weeks releasing them. I found that most people who came to me with CFIDS had a background similar to mine. They all seemed to manifest a very similar array of overgrowth. In fact, everyone had indications of systemic staph or strep, systemic candida, or ergot funguses, many types of viruses and parasites. Emotionally, they tended to be locked up inside and unable to experience their feelings. Many exhibited similar emotional patterns of depression, inability to focus and concentrate, inability to hold a job, and nervous system disorders. In many cases, there was a history of violent or abusive parents. Some had a history of drug usage and substance abuse. There were issues with self-esteem.

I developed a hypnosis program to assist them in releasing their emotional bodies. I was convinced that part of healing the immune system lay in healing the heart of old emotional wounds and opening up the feeling body. Some of my clients got better. Others did not. Most shared the same physical body experience: the overgrowth would gradually grow back after several months. This went on for several years. I was very frustrated. I knew I was close; I could eliminate the viruses and other overgrowth. The big question remained to be answered: why were they growing back?

I woke up one morning with new insight. I was missing something very important. It occurred to me that the bacteria, mycobacteria, viruses, funguses and para- sites might be "growing" on something else. I began to refer to this collection of parasitic vermin as "overgrowth" and began to look for something that was the basis of their life-force. I reasoned that if there were gases, and chemical substances that supported life and were the building blocks of cells and tissues, then there must be other chemicals and substances that support this family of "overgrowth" that was breaking down and destroying life. I began to identify this "overgrowth" as being the beginning of the process that breaks down cells and tis- sues upon death. For some reason, these vermin were feeding off of something in my body that was allowing them to systematically destroy my cells, even though I was not dead yet. Pretty eager characters!

THE CAUSE OF CHRONIC FATIGUE SYNDROME: Toxic Chemicals

November 12, 1990, I was drawn to a Time magazine article concerning the beaching and eventual death of striped dolphins, victims of pneumonia and liver damage, around the Mediterranean Sea. A viral epidemic of morbilli accounted for 50 deaths in a two-week period, bringing the total to 250 within three months. This virus is similar to the cause of canine distemper and human measles that killed some 20,000 North Sea seals in 1988. The article talked about the incredible pollution of the sea as a pos- sible cause of the problem. Autopsies showed dolphin tissues were contaminated with metals and toxic polychlorinated biphenyl's (PCPs).[7]

Could it be possible that humans and mammals were experiencing the same effects of our polluted environment? Could it be possible that the same thing that has been killing off dolphins in large numbers, might also be killing off humans in large numbers? Had the world gotten so polluted that all human life was dying off? I began to explore this possibility.

I started reading books on sources of pollution and testing for toxic chemicals in my body. I worked systematically for months. I developed long lists of common toxic substances and used the SE5 to help identify if I had residues of these toxins in my body. Much to my surprise, I was finding evidence of residues of many types of toxic substances. This included plutonium, strontium 90, long lists of pesticides, toxic solvents, herbicides, industrial solvents, heavy metals, and food preservatives. I was overwhelmed by the quantities and types of toxins in my subtle bodies. How could this be possible? How many more toxic chemicals were in my body? What was the source of this contamination? I had lots of questions. I wanted answers.

I developed my own theories and information concerning "residues" of toxic substances that remain in the body after they have been ingested.

Eventually, I decided that the "overgrowth" experienced by CFIDS and AIDS and other immune dysfunctional victims was growing on a base of toxic substances including, but not limited to, organophosphate pesticides, hydrocarbon solvents, food additives, drugs, poisons, alcohol, radioactive elements including plutonium and strontium 90, and toxic heavy metals.

CFIDS-SYMPTOMS OF DELAYED NEUROTOXICITY

My search for information led me to the book, **Chemical Deception** by Marc Lappe, that was to be a major key to my findings. In this book, Lappe talks about some of the history of the research involved with toxic chemicals and pesticides in this country.

I was drawn to a section in Chapter 5 in which he describes in detail the effects of "delayed neurotoxicity": the delayed effects of toxic substance poisonings. As I made notes on the symptoms of neurotoxicity, I became convinced that the symptoms that I had experienced with Chronic Fatigue Syndrome very closely resembled symptoms of toxic chemical poisoning.[8]

He states that early symptoms include tiredness, episodes of anxiety, loss of memory, confusion, irritability, depression, and sometimes vomiting as well. Long-term or progressed symptoms include impaired verbal abilities, defective psychomotor function, pervasive central nervous system damage, clinical depression, loss of ability to concentrate, short-term memory loss, inability to organize visual space, loss of color perception, loss of motor coordination, and pinpoint pupils.[9] The words "pinpoint pupils" jumped out at me from the page. My mind went quickly back to the practitioner who had told me that I had pinpoint pupils years before. As I looked at these symptoms, I realized that many of the symptoms listed right here accurately described the symptoms I had experienced in the past ten years of my life. Did this sound familiar? The bells started going off in my conscious mind. Perhaps I was really onto something.

Lappe goes on to list two general categories of toxic chemicals that cause delayed neurotoxicity effects in the body. The first category involves exposure to organo-phosphate esters, which are deadly nerve gas chemicals and pesticides. The second involves exposure to hydro-carbon solvents.

ORGANOPHOSPHATE ESTERS:
Pesticides & Nerve Gas Chemicals

I wanted to know what exactly organophosphate es-ters were and how one gets exposed to them.

Lappe defines organophosphorus esters as a group of phosphorus containing chemicals such as TOCP, triorothocresyl phosphate. The most deadly of chemi-cals, most have been developed since the 1930's. The majority of them have been developed since World War II. These esters are the principal components and by-products of chemical weapons, such as nerve gas and mustard gas. So lethal are these chemicals that normal doses are generally measured in milligrams. They are also used in the manufacture of pesticides which are extremely toxic.[10]

During 1993, Paris was the meeting place of repre-sentatives from over 100 nations world-wide, who negotiated and signed a complex treaty intended to ban the manufacture, stockpiling and use of chemical weapons. This treaty was considered one of the most complex arms control pacts ever negotiated because many of the same chemicals that are used in deadly weapons are also key ingredients of pesticides and other industrial products. For that reason, only a few lethal chemicals were outlawed by the treaty. Other compounds were placed under international supervision to prevent their diversion to military uses.[11]

For many, many years organophosphate chemicals have been involved with chemical warfare and part of the arsenals that the military and governments consider important to fighting wars. These chemicals are prized by those who would wage war because of their ability to inhibit the function of certain biological molecules. They are known as nerve gas chemicals. Since 1940, developers have tested over 500,000 organophosphate chemicals for pesticides and 200 or more of these chemicals have found their way into commercial use. The Environmental Protection Agency has at least 80 OP chemicals currently registered.

Organophosphate chemicals all have the ability to inhabit the production of the enzyme acetylcholinesterase, a key molecule needed to permit the regeneration of acetylcholine at neuromuscular junctions. This lack of acetylcholine interferes with nerve control of muscle transmissions. Someone poisoned by organophosphate pesticides will have low levels of acetylcholinesterase in their body and exhibit signs of chronic stimulation of certain muscle groups such as tearing, salivation, stomach cramps, vomiting and pinpoint pupils.[12]

I would also point out that lack of acetylcholinesterase has recently been indicated in newspaper articles as a possible cause of Alzheimer's disease.[13] This is, in fact, the property that makes them very effective as nerve gas chemicals that can kill soldiers and civilians after exposure to only a few drops. Tests with animals have shown that exposure to organophosphate compounds damages the central nervous system directly affecting the brain and spinal nerves. This nerve damage is generally irreversible.[14]

With time, the aging of OP pesticides produces changes in the chemicals which make them even more poisonous. Theoalkylphosphoryl is an extremely toxic chemical produced by this aging process. I often find it indicated in CFIDS clients. Although most of these chemicals are banned in the U.S., millions of pounds of them are sold to third world countries. Leptophose, Fenthion and Isophenthos are probably the most common types of Organophosphate Pesticides. More than seventeen million pounds of leptophose were marketed in 50 foreign countries between 1971 and 1976, in spite of indications of neurotoxicity findings in the U.S.[15] There are no laws prohibiting the importation of foods grown with these pesticides. As third world countries have grown more and more products for export, they have tried to increase exportable commodities by dumping larger and larger amounts of toxic pesticides on food products.

December 24, 1993, Moscow revealed that tens of

thousands of people had died who were involved with the production of chemical weapons in the former Soviet Union. The medical consequences of the production of chemical weapons was disastrous in that country. Estimates indicate that over 1 million people live in 300 towns in which chemical weapons were produced, stored, tested or destroyed. Today, these towns are highly contaminated areas where babies are born sick or abnormal in some way.

The results of the Soviet nuclear program are being felt by its citizens from one end of the union to the other. This secret program resulted in chemical pollution that has spoiled much of the ecology and threatens the health of its citizens. Factories that produced weapons during World War II offered no proper means of protection to its workers, dumped contaminated water into rivers, did not filter gas discharges, and burned lethal material like mustard gas at open sites. Today, a mustard gas production shop in Chapayevsk and an artillery shell production plant have two survivors each. The rest have died as a result of improper exposure to toxic poisons and gases. From 1924 to the mid 1980's, toxic chemicals and nuclear waste were dumped into the Baltic, Barents and Beloye Seas off Russia's northern coast, the Far Eastern seas of Japan and Okhotsk and other coastal waters without any concern for the consequences.[16]

Something tells me that when all is known, our military record regarding chemical weapons will not be any better. What has come to light to date would indicate that a very similar philosophy has prevailed in the U.S.

The January signing of the treaty to ban chemical weapons was a major step in the right direction. I urge the members of the same nations to take another look at the facts and consider the possibility that the same chemicals in pesticides might also have serious effects on thousands, perhaps millions of people. We must care about the safety of our planet and our most valuable resource – people. We must all work together to clean up this world for ourselves and for our children.

HYDROCARBON SOLVENTS:
Industrial Pollution

Exposure to hydrocarbon solvents is the other major source of "delayed neurotoxicity" poisoning. Solvents are a major part of the technological information age that we live in today. The first major source of hydrocarbon pollution is industry. Large chemical companies and industrial manufacturers have encountered major problems in today's world. Oil spills, chemical spills, and chemical pollution are very large headaches faced on a daily basis by companies like Exxon, Union Carbide and IBM.

Solvents are used in the production of, or are main components of, almost everything that we take for granted. This includes oil, gasoline, paint, computer chips, TV's, VCR's, telephones, fabric, glue, paper, cleaning products, plastic, fertilizers, etc., etc. Just about everything we have come to rely upon in our daily life has some connection to industrial solvents.

October, 1992. IBM warned its workers that two

chemicals widely used in manufacturing semiconductor chips may increase the risk of miscarriage. The chemicals were identified as diethylene glycol dimethl ether and ethylene glycol monethyl ether acetate. [17]

June, 1992. Environmental contaminants, particularly PCBs and pesticide by-products, were for the first time linked to breast cancer in humans. Hartford Hospital studies indicated that fatty breast tissue from women with malignant breast tumors contained more than twice as much PCBs (polychlorinated biphenyl's) and DDEs (dichlorodiphenyldichloro-ethylene) as were found in the breast fat of women of the same age and weight who did not have cancer. [18]

March, 1989. The Exxon Valdez spilled 11 million gallons of crude oil into Alaska's Prince William Sound, in what was considered the worst oil spill in history. [19]

December 1992. The Greek tanker, Aegean Sea, lost 21.5 million gallons of crude oil off the coast of Spain. No one knows for sure the impact this type of spills will have on fish and shellfish in the waters. Officials estimated at least $15 million damage from ruined mussel farms, spoiled shellfish beds and wrecked equipment. What about the buildup of toxins in humans from eating sea life that survived the initial spill, but contain high residue levels from these toxic chemicals? [20]

December 1993. Officials trying to get a navigable path cleared through the Ashtabula River in Northeast Ohio, ponder what to do with the muck contaminated with heavy metals and cancer causing chemicals. The government built 26 places around the Great Lakes to hold dredged-out mud too polluted to dump back into the water. It is estimated that by the year 2006, 24 of 26 facilities will be filled. Five million cubic yards of silt are dredged out of the Great Lakes each year. Contaminated mud was routinely dumped back into the lake until Congress decided that the soil should be dumped elsewhere. Congress assumed that the flow of pollution would stop in ten years, but new pollutants keep turning up in the lakes.[21]

As early as 1956, studies appeared indicating long-term toxic effects in humans from many of the solvents common to industrial usage and manufacture. Much of the research initially linking hydrocarbon solvents with dis-ease and cancer was repressed. There seemed to be no common meeting of the minds as to how much exposure would result in dysfunction or dis-ease, so the problem was largely ignored.[22] Perhaps this had something to do with the power and influence of the companies manufacturing these toxic chemicals and solvents. This was BIG business, literally millions, perhaps billions, of dollars were involved. These manufacturers had lots of money to lobby for their special interests. As a result, all citizens have been placed on the brink of a genetic breakdown that could affect every aspect of our lives. Perhaps our very species will disappear. This is not science fiction. This is reality for the 1990's. Manufacturers must change their thinking or we are in real trouble. We must work together for change. We don't have time for blame.

Symptoms one might experience from exposure to hydrocarbon solvents include loss of memory, slowing of intellectual processes, sleep disorder, disorientation and emotional instability, blurred vision, damage to motor and sensory nerves, loss of appetite, fatigue, headaches, weight loss, altered color perception, impaired verbal ability, defective psychomotor function, dementia, clinical depression, insomnia, and profound central nervous system damage.[23]

THE MILITARY'S ROLE:
Hydrocarbon Pollution

The military is the other major source of environmental pollution by hydrocarbon solvents. The Pentagon produces well over a ton of toxic wastes every minute. Most people do not realize that the military complex has operated almost entirely unrestricted by environmental law. The military operates by a much different set of rules and routinely sanctions practices illegal for private industry. Billions of gallons of toxic wastes have been dumped directly into the ground at thousands of sites across the world for decades. The Pentagon has done its best to keep the dumping secret, and by its actions has threatened the health and welfare not only of Americans, but all of earth's citizens. [24]

The results of the actions and attitudes of our war mentality have caught up with us. The types of lethal toxic waste inherent to all military operations worldwide may someday be indicated as a major underlying cause of many diseases and disorders. This includes nuclear waste, chemical weapons, and other lethal toxic solvents.

Much information has come to light in recent months concerning the contamination of military bases in California. Many of the bases being closed are also SUPER-FUND SITES which will require many millions of dollars and perhaps years to clean up. Perhaps we will never truly know the full extent of the military's role in worldwide pollution. The price of the military industrial complex, the nuclear arsenals and all the weapons to wage war has been probably more than the earth can truly afford.

We are not the only country responsible for lethal toxic pollution. Recent news articles indicate that the former Soviet Union had been dumping radioactive wastes in the oceans for years. When the truth is known, I am sure that all countries with active military complexes will have to take the blame for what has been created.

THE PHILIPPINE LEGACY

After 40 years of occupying bases on the Philippine Islands, the U.S. troops left behind quite a remembrance. Notably a legacy of stored and improperly disposed of military and industrial wastes on and around Subic Naval Base and Clark Air Base. This included: 1) improper storage and use of hazardous materials banned in the U.S., such as asbestos and polychlorinated biphenyl or PCBs; 2) thousands of gallons of highly corrosive aviation fuel left behind in an underground pipeline stretching between the two bases; 3) live bombs and ammunition; 4) lead and heavy metals dumped into Subic Bay; 5) over 300 barrels of toxic chemicals, including acids and solvents abandoned in an open field; 6) toxic chemicals poured into open drains and used underground fuel storage tanks without proper leak detection equipment. Subic generated more than 500 tons of hazardous waste a year, but disposed of less that 20 percent.[25]

There is no reason to believe that the bases in the Philippines are any different from other military bases. So multiply this times the hundreds of installations around the world, regardless of which flag flies over the installation. As you can readily see, it is truly a worldwide problem experienced by every nation on the earth today.

AFTERMATH: THE PERSIAN GULF WAR

The aftermath of the Persian Gulf War has left hundreds of veterans with ailments that baffle doctors. Scores of Persian Gulf vets have complained about mysterious symptoms since returning from the Middle East. Complaints include Chronic Fatigue, strange rashes, respiratory problems, achey joints, bleeding gums and hair loss. The Veterans Affairs Agency thinks problems could have been caused by smoke, contaminated food or drink, burning oil wells, or environmental conditions.[26]

First let me say, that all of these symptoms are on the list of common CFIDS symptoms that I have listed in the back of this book. There are several things that come to mind here. Any one, or a combination of all, could be at work. I would not know for sure without an opportunity to analyze a hair sample which would allow me to identify residues of toxins present.

The first intuitive hit would be that these veterans are suffering from exposure to chemical warfare nerve gas. Who is to say that Iraq did not install nerve gas containers in the scudd missiles that were so artfully shot down by the U.S. technical weapons. Explosion of the scudd missiles could release the nerve gas chemicals into the air and soil for all to breathe. The second possibility is exposure to plutonium radiation. I don't really know much about war and nuclear weapons, but there may be several possible sources indicated here. One could be from our own arsenal of weapons employed in the Gulf War. Perhaps there are other avenues of exposure as well.

Personally, I do not think that we will ever fully know all the kinds and types of technological weapons that were tested in this war. Radiation and radioactive fallout remain a strong possibility in my mind. The third source of contamination could be from smoke inhalation from the burning oil fields. Finally, we need to look at food and water supplies. They could be contaminated with pesticides and/or radiation or other toxic materials. Accumulated residues from any one of these chemical toxins could produce the effects reported by veterans. I am sure there could be many more toxic chemicals involved as well. War is a toxic game.

In his book, **The Threat At Home**, Seth Shulman describes in detail the types of contamination the military has left at bases and installations on U.S. soil. He identifies the types of toxic pollution likely to be found at the different bases, and identifies those designated as

SUPERFUND SITES. He describes in detail some of the chemicals that are unique to the military designed to serve exclusive military purposes which are outlawed in private industry because of the lethal toxicity. This includes solvents, like Decontamination Solution #2, or DS2, that can cause central nervous system depression, liver damage and birth defects. It will eat through metal, rubber, human skin and tissue. A highly corrosive compound described by the military as "nasty stuff", little health data exists. It is stockpiled in almost every Army base in the U.S. and abroad. [27]

Other toxic substances include solvents, such as Research and Development Explosive, RDX, (hexahydro-1,3,5-trinitro-1,3,5-triazine); Dinitrotoluene, DNT; and trinitrotoluene, TNT, which are natural by-products of the manufacture of ammunitions and are found as a major components of "toxic red water". These explosive compounds have found their way into many water supplies in cities, counties and states in the U.S. and around the world. U.S. Public Health Service's Agency for Toxic Substances and Disease Registry studies have linked these chemicals to nervous system disorders, kidney damage, and liver cancer. [28]

People who live in and around military bases, including ammunition manufacturing bases, and nuclear storage sites should be alarmed and concerned about contamination levels of their water, soil, and air. I feel that many communities have, unknowingly, been subject to dangerous levels of toxins in their drinking water and soil. Perhaps the time has come for all citizens to purify or filter their tap water. Water needs to be screened for all types of toxic substances. Local governments and civillians must work with the military to identify and solve this problem. We have the technology to turn this around.

I cannot help noticing that certain areas in California are experiencing extreme problems with violence and drugs are located close to major military bases or toxic chemical plants. Some of this may be due to drug influence. I wonder how much of this violence can be attributed to the presence of residues of lethal chemicals in the water, food, and air. I wonder about the statistics concerning CFIDS, AIDS and Alzheimer's in these areas.

The Defense Reutilization and Marketing Service is the agency which handles military surplus. Toxic military chemicals can be purchased at auctions handled by this agency, which receives more than 150 million pounds of hazardous wastes every year. In 1989, the DRMS disposed of 106 million pounds of wastes. However the destination of 72 million pounds of toxic wastes received that year are unclear. They were perhaps sold, donated, or recycled.[29] We have a major problem on our hands. We have run out of space to safely dispose of toxic waste. We need creative alternatives.

It is a normal practice of the defense department to include unwanted toxic materials in mixed lots of supplies sold to the public. If you wanted to purchase some office equipment, desks or typewriters, they might throw in some barrels of toxic chemicals as well. [30] Since they have no civilian use, one wonders how many barrels of toxic materials ended up along the roadside, illegally dumped in lakes or buried in someone's vacant lot. People have had to be very creative in unloading this stuff. Some have simply been stored in warehouses or deserted buildings with the hope that they would go undiscovered.

The list of toxic substances includes herbicides, mustard gases, nerve gases, special purpose solvents, toxic red water, radioactive wastes, and waste oils, heavy metals, acids, cyanide, trichlorethylene, aviation fuels, polychlorinated biphenyl's, and oil and gas spillage from ruptured under ground storage tanks.[31] I suggest that you read **The Threat at Home**; it is very frightening.

RADIATION

Radiation is another major factor involved with CFIDS and other immune dysfunction disease. I noticed early in my research that people who came to me with CFIDS often had high levels of radiation in their bodies. This included high levels of plutonium and strontium 90 and radioactive fallout. My first reaction was disbelief. How could that be? Plutonium is very deadly. Where could this be coming from?

I soon discovered that clients with high levels of radiation also had low levels of calcium in their subtle bodies. I began to notice that if you added the two levels together, they would total 100%. Was there a correlation between high levels of radiation and calcium in the body? I casually mentioned this discovery to a friend and client. She replied, "Yes, indeed this was true." She went on to say that her father was a chemist involved in major research on this subject in the 1940's. He was dead now, but perhaps she could get me a copy of his research. Unfortunately, that was not to be.

I started scanning the bookstores looking for information. I found several books on the subject. There is, in fact, a relationship between certain types of radiation and calcium. This includes Cesium 137 and Strontium 90. The molecular structure is so similar to calcium that the body does not seem to be able to tell the difference.[32] It thinks it has all the calcium it needs and will not digest any more. This is probably why I was still calcium-deficient even though I had been taking supplements and digestive enzymes for years now. This is why my teeth were breaking. I wondered if this was also the cause of osteoporosis in older people. It seems important to mention that the government wants to use Cesium 137 to irradiate meat and cattle products to eliminate the bacteria that has become a problem. I strongly suggest that this not be done.

INDEPENDENT RESEARCH ON RADIATION EXPOSURE

The first independent study of health records of 35,000 workers at the Hanford, Washington, bomb plant indicates that exposure to small doses of radiation are much more dangerous than the government would like for us to believe. For decades the government controlled access to health data and limited this access to scientists who concluded that radiation exposure had little to no harmful effects on those plant workers exposed.

Dr. Alice Steward recently concluded the first independent study of health data and came to very different conclusions. Her studies showed that 200 of the workers have lost, or will lose, years of their lives because of radiation-induced cancer. Her results are contradictory to government-sponsored studies which found no additional cancer deaths among the employees. Dr. Steward concluded that low doses of radiation had caused an increase in the number of cancers developed over the years. Other conclusions are: 1) Even small doses of radiation are four to eight times more likely to cause cancer than previously believed. 2) People are far more vulnerable to radiation-induced cancer if the exposure comes later in life. 3) Radiation delivered in small doses over time may carry a higher risk of cancer than radiation delivered in a single dose. The current consensus is that small doses of the most common form of radiation are less damaging because the body has time to repair itself. [33]

It would seem that the government has not been honest with us concerning the danger of radiation. I wonder why?

Let's take a look at information that is available to us concerning the former Soviet Union's romance with atomic energy.

NUCLEAR LEGACY IN FORMER SOVIET UNION

We know that the USSR conducted many secret nuclear tests. Articles indicate that the USSR subjected citizens and soldiers alike to unnecessary nuclear fallout on several occasions. Over the years, more than 100 nuclear bombs were detonated for "peaceful purposes" across the vast terrain of the former Soviet Union. An estimated 20 million Soviets were exposed to radioactivity released at Chernobyl. Millions of others received doses from bomb tests at Semipalatinsk and Novaya Zemlya in the Arctic, sometimes as intentional guinea pigs. Yellow children born in Talmenka, Russia, were classified as "nuclear mutants", the most recent victims of nuclear technology.

High-level radioactive waste was routinely dumped into lakes and rivers, even those used as sources of drinking water. Large population bases like Moscow and St. Petersburg were fouled by dump sites for nuclear waste. Moscow, home to more than 9 million people, has at least 600 secret waste dumps whose radiation levels are dangerously high.

A once-secret weapons-grade plutonium plant near Chelyabinsk in the southern Urals has accumulated so much radioactive waste that if spread evenly over the former Soviet Union, there would be enough to poison every square foot. The accumulated waste is stored in open lakes, dumps and storage pools. Both long and short term effects on human health seem tragic. The nuclear wastes left by the Soviet military are permanent scars on that continent, and will be there for a very long time.[34]

What a tragic situation. Before we sit back and "thank God" we do not live in the Soviet Union, it is important that we take a closer look at our own situation. The DOE has recently admitted similar testing.

SECRET NUCLEAR PROGRAM IN UNITED STATES OF AMERICA

In December, 1993, the U.S. Department of Energy admitted that it conducted hundreds of secret nuclear tests, far beyond those that had been reported to the public. This includes 204 secret nuclear blasts in Nevada between 1963 and 1990. The DOE admits that thirty seven of these tests released radioactivity into the atmosphere. Lawrence Livermore Laboratory conducted 97 of the tests. The DOE also conducted 800 radiation tests on humans, including injecting civilians with highly radioactive plutonium in the 1940's.

The same report indicates that the U.S. produced nearly 200,000 pounds of weapons-grade plutonium between 1945 and 1988. Plutonium is without a doubt the most toxic, deadly material ever produced on earth. The Department of Energy lists stockpiles of plutonium around the country including Richland, Washington; Lawrence Livermore National Lab, California; Los Alamos, New Mexico; Rocky Flats, Colorado; Idaho National Engineering Lab, Idaho; Argonne National Lab-West, Idaho; Pantex,

Texas; and Savannah River, South Carolina.[35]

Questions arise in my mind about the connection to high levels of plutonium found in CFIDS clients and the secret activities of the Department of Energy. My first questions is "what has the government done with all the wastes that would be involved with the production of weapons-grade plutonium?" If the Soviet experience is typical, I would say that there is a huge amount of toxic waste that has been stored and dumped. Would you suspect that our government might be dumping and disposing of this waste in ways that might prove to be extremely detrimental to our health and that of our children? This is a serious situation that requires immediate action, as we cannot afford to let this happen.

Shulman goes into great detail about the problems encountered at Hanford Nuclear Reservation, in Richland, Washington, with disposal and storage of toxic uranium and nuclear waste in his book, **The Threat At Home.** The problems and costs involved with clean up of over 30 million cubic feet of nuclear waste and close to 100 times that in radiated soil are staggering. The big concern should be the radioactive ground water which leaked through underground storage tanks and has found its way into the Columbia River six miles away. Indications are that radioactive strontium 90 has contaminated the river with up to 500 times the amount considered safe by federal standards.[36] One wonders what other types of radiation and toxic solvents are floating down the river into our taps on a daily basis. Or perhaps the water is irrigating the farm lands which grow our food supplies.

Are you listening, folks? The Columbia River is a major source of water for Washington, Oregon, and California.

POINT HOPE, ALASKA

In 1962, the Inupiat Eskimos successfully stopped a plan by the federal government to create an Arctic harbor with a huge atomic blast near the village of Point Hope. Undaunted, the U.S. government proceeded to secretly bury several thousand pounds of radioactive soil outside the village near Point Hope, on the Chukchi Sea in northwestern Alaska. The soil contained trace amounts of fallout from a nuclear explosion at the Nevada Test Site and was part of a project designed to study how radioactivity spreads in an Arctic environment. The site was unmarked. Nothing was done to warn the villages of this action, or the possible dangers of it. Natives of the North Slope have a cancer rate that far exceeds the national average.[37]

The question arises as to what other locations may have been involved in this secret project? Where else have they disposed of this radioactive waste? Alaska might be a prize choice because of the small population base. Is there any connection here to my developing CFIDS and my dog developing similar symptoms? We lived very close to Fort Richardson military base in Alaska at that time.

The second question that comes to mind involves radioactive fallout from these tests. We are all aware of the fallout associated with the Chernobyl explosion in April, 1986. Ukrainian doctors routinely refer to what they call "Chernobyl AIDS", a radiation-caused immune deficiency that is not understood, or even accepted, by the medical community. A mixed bag of illnesses, including pneumonia, tuberculosis, vision problems such as cataracts, anemia and other blood disorders, headaches, sleeplessness, nosebleeds and hair loss are all on the rise. (Do any of these symptoms sound like CFIDS or AIDS?) Radiation damage to living cells is slow acting and may take years to manifest on the physical level. Although tumors and leukemia might take years to develop after initial exposures, the radiation will genetically determine disorders that appear in the next generation. The government's response to this is one of denial and neglect. There is a huge gulf between symptoms people are experiencing and what officials say they should be experiencing.[38]

On December 16, 1993, the Department of Energy further revealed that between 1948 and 1952, the U.S. government deliberately dropped radioactive material from planes or released it on the ground in a dozen experiments. Eight of the tests occurred in Tennessee and Utah and were part of an experiment to create a battlefield radiation weapon. In an attempt to plot its movements, pilots chased radiation deliberately released over New Mexico on four different occasions. In other tests, radiation spread beyond the planned boundaries of the test.[39]

I was between five and nine years old at the time, living in Louisville, Kentucky which is very close to Tennessee. Could it be possible that I was exposed to radiation from one of these

94

tests, along with thousands, possibly millions, of others? I wonder if my father was injected in some secret Navy program during the war, or exposed to radiation through some other military source? Could this be the source of his mysterious illness that stumped the doctors? What is incidence of CFIDS and cancer in these areas?

In 1949, experiments spread radiation over a 200 mile stretch of Oregon and Washington state. In tests designed to demonstrate how radioactive clouds disperse, radiation bombs were dropped from planes over Los Alamos, New Mexico. The release created radioactive clouds that were traced 10 miles in one case, 70 miles in another. In other tests, the distance traveled by the clouds was unknown. In Utah, radiation bombs dropped at an Army site spread 50% farther than expected.

In the fall of 1949, the Army dropped cluster bombs containing radiation particles reaching 1500 curies from a plane flying at 15,000 feet. That level of radiation could cause death to those exposed at extremely close range in about an hour.

A curie is a measure of radioactivity equal to the amount of radiation produced by a gram of radium. The Three Mile Island emergency emitted no more than 15 curies of radiation. The above tests performed by our government emitted radioactive levels from 300 to 1500 curies. Experts claim that the radiation would have dispersed relatively quickly, and that no radioactive residues would remain in those areas today.[40]

Do you believe this? The government has not exactly been truthful to its citizens concerning its nuclear program. Something in me does not buy this. Neither do the populations in some of the remote communities down-wind from the experimental sites. It is not the nature of radiation to disperse quickly. Plutonium has a half-life of 24,000 years. We all know of the contamination of communities in Europe and Belorussia from radiation released from the Chernobyl incident.

What about the long term effects of plutonium build up in humans from continued exposure to water supplies and soil that may have been contaminated with radiation fallout from these tests? That would also apply to the cattle and other animals. If exposure to large amounts of radiation can cause AIDS-like symptoms, it would seem possible that long term exposure to small amounts of radiation might result in a watered-down version of AIDS, such as CFIDS.

One must also look at the genetic damage that would be passed on to children of citizens exposed to radiation from these tests. I have a strong sense that these might also be CFIDS sufferers of today. What will tomorrow bring?

INCLINE VILLAGE

In Incline Village, Nevada, 1984 saw an outbreak of "flu" virus in over 200 of the Village's 20,000 residents. Trouble was, unlike the flu, no one seemed to get better. Local doctors Paul Cheney and Daniel Peterson grew alarmed about the situation when tests indicated that sufferers were mass-producing anti-bodies to Epstein-Barr virus, a herpes virus involved with mononucleosis. He reported the situation to the Center for Disease Control when additional blood tests showed indications of herpes simplex and cytomegalovirus.

In 1986, Dr. David Bell read about the situation in Incline Village. He saw some parallels to the mysterious symptoms experienced by his patients who were plagued with a strange flu-like illness which left them with enlarged spleens and swollen lymph nodes. Most of his patients were children living in Lyndonville, NY. In a short time his patient load had grown to 30 children and adults. Attempts to enlist help from the state health department failed. His own survey turned up a few common threads including 1) those stricken had a history of allergies; 2) several families had more than one member afflicted; 3) several families seemed to have been drinking unpasteurized milk: two families were drinking milk from the same goat. Could the milk be contaminated?

In 1987 with his caseload still growing, Dr. Bell came across a patient with all the classic symptoms of this Lyndonville syndrome, only she was from Southern California. He knew then that this was the same dis-ease that the Lake Tahoe doctors were struggling with. Other doctors became involved. Research indicated that this was an organic illness.

Portland, Oregon was the site of the first conference on Chronic Fatigue Syndrome. The year was 1987. Doctors came from all parts of the U.S. to compare notes. Other viruses were being added to the Epstein-Barr virus, including herpes HHV-6, polio, coxsackie, and ocho.

Tests showed these viruses were active in some patients, but none were active in all—quite a mystery. The doctors did agree that Chronic Fatigue Syndrome was an immune disorder. A doctor from So. California theorized that the illness begins when "Agent x" enters and damages the immune system. "Agent x" was most likely an unknown chemical or contagion. To date scientists have not been successful in attempts to identify "Agent x".[41]

I would strongly suspect that the cause of the initial outbreak of CFIDS in the small resort town of Incline Village in the fall of 1984, as well as outbreaks in Lydonville, NY, will eventually be linked to radiation exposure either from fallout (from DOE's nuclear testing) or some nuclear dump site in the area which has contaminated water supplies.

I cannot help but wonder if there was a nuclear test that might coincide with the Incline Village incident. We need to seriously consider that possibility. How can we be sure there are not nuclear waste dump sites near these towns or major cities as well? This seems to be the case in the former Soviet Union.

VIRUS KILLING DEER IN CALIFORNIA

Recent newspaper articles indicate that there have been 20 mysterious deer deaths in a 2 mile radius of Sonora, a little Mother lode town in the western slopes of the Sierra Nevada. Wild deer began dropping dead by the hundreds throughout Northern California in late July, 1993 signaling a massive die-off of animals in a short period of time. Death toll is believed to be in the thousands. A DNA-mutating strain of virus (adenovirus), never encountered before turned out to be the culprit. Adenoviruses are a broad category of infectious viruses that spread like cancer, altering DNA and causing respiratory disease. Indications are that the virus had lingered dormant in the deer population since 1987. The high Sierra towns in Tuolumne and Nevada counties show signs that the deer populations might be decimated in these areas.[42]

I would suspect that the deer are the victims of radioactive fallout or toxic nuclear waste. I suggest that those investigating this virus look for indications of radiation poisoning. The area around Sonora should be investigated for dangerous toxic waste sites, including nuclear wastes. This area is close enough to the Nevada test site to have received hefty doses of radiation from the recently admitted 204 secret nuclear tests. It would not hurt to check it out. You might be surprised at the findings.

<u>December, 1992</u>. Kern Country, California, reported an epidemic of Valley Fever, a strange dust-borne disease endemic to the Southwest, infecting more than 4000 people and killing 34. The incidence of Valley Fever has exploded tenfold since the summer of 1991 and shows no sign of abating. Kern County cases account for two-thirds of the cases and deaths statewide. The disease has also afflicted record numbers in Los Angeles, Ventura, Santa Barbara, Tulare and San Luis Obispo counties. At least 6000 people statewide have been infected with the

99

fungus found in the arid soils of Central and Southern California, Arizona, New Mexico and Texas. The fungus that causes Valley Fever is known by the name Coccidioides Immitis. People who work closely with the soil-construction and oil workers, land graders, farm workers and college students on archeological digs rank among the groups most afflicted. [43]

My intuition says to look for radiation exposure here as well. Once again, the soil may have been contaminated by nuclear fallout, or nuclear waste dump sites. Any of these areas could have experienced radioactive fallout from nearby Nevada Testing Grounds. Perhaps the fungus is blowing in from the desert. The desert would be a good place to store or hide nuclear waste. So would mountainous areas with small populations. New Mexico was one of the sites listed by the DOE where weapons grade plutonium is stored. How many other places exist that may have been targets of the nuclear program that have not been identified? How many other tests are unreported?

December, 1993. Information has come to light indicating that 200 babies in five states were intentionally injected with radioactive iodine during government experiments in the 1950's and 1960's. The latest disclosures on nuclear research indicated that tests were performed in Tennessee, Michigan, Nebraska, Arkansas and Iowa. The fate of these infants is unknown as no follow-up work was ever done.

Between 1951 and 1975, human experiments were supported by the Atomic Energy Commission, NASA, and the U.S. Public Health Service. Researchers injected people with phosphorus-32, radioactive technitium, or promethium as well as radioactive iron and chrome.[44]

TRAVIS AIR FORCE BASE CRASH

<u>February 18, 1994</u>. Air Force officials have recently admitted that a B-29 that crashed at Travis Air Force Base in 1950 carried secret cargo including an "unarmed atom bomb" and 100 pounds of radioactive uranium. Rob Heitmann's efforts to uncover information concerning his son's diagnosis of leukemia eventually lead to the discovery of this well kept military secret. Rob's suspicion that his son's cancer might somehow be connected to Travis Elementary School resulted in over three years of frustrating research into the history of toxic chemicals at Travis. Much to his surprise, he learned about the crash and atom bomb which killed 19 people on board and left a crater 20 yards wide and 6 feet deep on the runway. He also learned that the elementary school was built on the crash site.

Air Force sources claim that the plane did not carry the nuclear core and as a consequence, there was little concern for the depleted uranium that was aboard—it could cause few long-term health problems. Heitmann's concern for other children attending the school and residents of Vacaville lead him to release the information to the Vacaville Reporter. Officials have agreed to analyze the soil for traces of radioactive material.[45]

When governments keep secrets from their citizens,

a credibility gap is the result. Can we really believe what the government is telling us the truth about this incident? What else are they keeping secret? What would have been the long term effects if there was a nuclear core aboard that plane and it went off? How much land would have been contaminated? What long-term effect would this have had? Were there other secret crashes? I think we have the right to know.

How many other people are unknowing victims of this secret nuclear research? I bet every CFIDS sufferer in the U.S. is going to wonder if he or she was injected with radiation by our government at the time of their birth, or during other medical procedures. I know that I certainly do. We have the right to ask that question. Radiation can cause CFIDS, cancer and leukemia. Permission was not asked. No warning or indication was given to the parents or children. No follow up was done. How heartless can the government be? Can this be compared to the type of research that was done in Nazi Germany? How many other secret programs have yet to be discovered? How many people have lost their lives because of the secrets they learned? To what extent has our government gone to protect their secret programs? We, as free citizens, need to think again about the privileges of living in a free country. We as a nation need to question our deepest fears and insecurities which created this situation.

I feel it is important to applaud the actions of Department of Energy Secretary, Hazel O'Leary, for her fortitude and courage in making this information public over objections of many. Also, applause needs to go to

Senator John Glenn, D-Ohio, chairman of the Committee of Governmental Affairs, who is behind the investigations of the nuclear weapons industry.

I hope that you will join me in a united voice of the people that will not rest until all of the secret story is told in full and all actions against America's citizens are accounted for. The back of this book contains a form letter that can be sent to your representatives voicing your concern and interest in this project. Take a moment to let your feelings be known. Get involved in this matter. It is important that we, the citizens of the U.S., let our government know how we feel about the secret nuclear testing and what we can do to make sure it does not happen in the future. It is time for us to wake up and take full responsibility for what we have created, then take action to turn it around. We need to ask the question: HOW CAN THIS HAPPEN IN A FREE COUNTRY WHERE THERE IS GOVERNMENT BY THE PEOPLE AND FOR THE PEOPLE AS OUR CONSTITUTION GUARANTEES? WHAT HAS GONE WRONG HERE? The answer lies inside of us. To change the world we must first change our own thinking.

The question remains, when are we going to find out the full truth regarding the U.S. military-industrial complex and our nuclear testing program? The truth needs to be known. We must act swiftly to begin a massive cleanup effort so we can reverse what has already been started. We must take affirmative action to set up clinics to assist people who already show symptoms of immune dysfunction diseases. We must join together in a worldwide effort to aid sufferers. The alternative will mean massive population die-off.

Can we believe the information that has recently come to light is the whole truth as well? In order to restore trust and cooperation among nations, we must first re-store trust within our own country. It is time to take a hard look at where we stand. We must know the truth.

REVERSING THE MAGNETIC POLES

We need to take a look at what actually happens in a nuclear reaction, or the process that makes a substance radioactive. During this process, the magnetic force that "glues" the atoms, molecules and subatomic particles together gets reversed. This "glue" is often called life force, or "love" energy in metaphysical terms, and is generated by the clockwise spin of molecules. When the fields get reversed, these atoms, molecules and subatomic particles actually become repulsed from each other. The electrons spinning around the molecules shoot off in an erratic pattern and the molecules start coming apart and break-ing down. Actually, this counter-clockwise spin is present in all toxic chemicals and substances that do not support life.

As world governments continue to detonate nuclear bombs and nuclear reactors are used to produce energy, what is actually happening on a world-wide level is that the magnetic force that creates and holds life together is getting destroyed. Slowly, the atoms, molecules, and sub-atomic particles are broken down. As our air, our food atomic particles are broken down. As our air, our food and water supplies are contaminated by radioactive substances, these residues build up in the cells of our bodies. As they invade the cells, they start a chain reaction of breaking down and reversing the spin in the subatomic particles of the cells. As residue levels accumulate in the body, the atoms and molecules start breaking down. As the magnetic force gets reversed in the bodies, the cells literally begin to fall apart and disintegrate. If these toxic substances include trace amounts of extremely toxic solvents that will literally "melt the flesh", you have a problem with a lot of dying people.

This seems to be one of the characteristics of a retrovirus. It breaks down the cell membrane and the cell literally starts falling apart. If the substances that really break the cells down are toxic chemicals, including caustic solvents and radioactive elements, you can see why traditional medicine has been unable to solve or cure this problem.

When you introduce nuclear technology into a planet, you accelerate the "aging" process of the planet, creating the vehicle that will begin to take it into the backside of a life cycle which is a death cycle. You introduce the means by which the forces that provide the life force necessary for human life to exist begin to break down. As a result, all life starts dying in mass quantities.

RESIDUES

I have mentioned in several places that I have developed my own theory concerning the breakdown of toxic chemicals in the body. Popular attitudes by scientists and toxicologists hold to the idea that toxic substances can only damage the body while they are present in the body. They do not seem to understand that residues of toxic chemicals will stay in the body for months, or years before they break down. Scientists seem unaware that residues of these substances can build up and accumulate in the tissues of the body.

My research indicates that residues of toxic chemical solvents, pesticides, drugs, alcohol, radioactive materials, and heavy metals remain in the body and may take years to break down. Just as DDT residues have been found in the water and soil years after they have been banned from usage, the same thing holds true for the human body.

Residue levels will accumulate and build up in the tissues and cells of the body. Once the tissues are saturated, these residues will float around in the blood stream, clogging blood vessels and arteries. It is my opinion that residues of toxic chemicals are the cause of cholesterol in the blood and plaque on the teeth, as well as CFIDS, AIDS, cancers, Alzheimer's and probably most other diseases as well. Anyone who has ever had their teeth cleaned knows how hard plaque is to remove from teeth. Residues form a white crystalline powder, which will stick together creating a very cement-like matter that will clog the blood vessels, arteries, and glands of the body. Residues will also be stored in the fatty tissues of the body.

Residues will accumulate in the arteries and blood vessels of the brain reducing the blood flow to part of the brain. They will clog veins and arteries in other organs as well, including the kidneys and liver, and build up on intestinal walls. I feel it is the tendency of residues to crystallize together in a concrete-like mass that is the underlying cause of the inflammation and irregular brain function attributed to CFIDS and AIDS patients. Remember that bacteria such as staph and strep grow off toxic chemicals. This same phenomenon also occurs in Alzheimer's disease. Perhaps there are different types of chemicals involved in Alzheimer's, CFIDS, and AIDS, but the underlying cause is the same. I am confident that time and more research will show this to be a fact.

It was only about a year and a half ago I had a clairvoyant Reiki practitioner, who was also my roommate in Maui, first indicate the presence of this "concrete-like mass" in my brain. She indicated that channeling Reiki energy into the mass started to break it up. However, much more work was needed. Neither one of us knew the source of the substance, or, how it got there. Shortly after my experience in the Reiki session, something happened that brought information to light concerning the origin and composition of this mass.

The first thing that happened was that I began to have nightmares involving a Black man who was a rapist and drug addict. I was very disturbed by these recurring dreams. As a hypnotherapist, I spent a lot of time releasing entities, spirit forms, on other dimensions. In the beginning, I assumed that this was an entity that I had picked up, perhaps from a client. But it did not act like an entity.

I enlisted the help of a psychic who concluded that this was a person whose blood I had received during the birth of my youngest son. I learned during this time that when you receive blood from another person, you become "fused" with that energy on other dimensions. In fact, you will take on that person's "karma" so to speak. As a result of the blood transfusion, this Black man became a part of my life, and I took on all the energy and "karma" that he had created. This included the drugs, and the energy of a sexual rapist. All I could say was, "what a journey!" No wonder my life changed and things got really intense. Besides all the sickness I was going through, much of it caused by the drugs and toxic chemicals I had taken into my body by the blood transfusion, I also had been dealing with all the other energy of a rapist. No wonder I could not manifest a loving man in my life. Just the thought of all this overwhelmed me. I realized that if I had known this from the beginning, I would have given up a long time ago.

The psychic indicated that much of the crystallized white mass in my brain was related to the drugs I inherited in the blood transfusion. Upon discovering the presence of this energy, and the situation, I worked with the psychic healer to separate the "fusion" and remove him from my energy field. Shortly after, I began researching the type of drug residues that were present in my brain, and worked with the SE5 to eliminate them.

I reasoned that if the person I received a blood transfusion from had been a drug user, and if my theories concerning "residues" were correct, then I should find drug residues in my body. I did not know much about drugs. So, I set out to do research as I had often done before. I went to my local bookstore and started looking for a comprehensive guide to the types of drugs available on the streets. I wanted to know if I could add drugs to the growing list of toxic chemical residues present in my body. I purchased several books, including ones listing the names of common street drugs, hallucinogenic plants, and prescription drugs.

I set about with my SE5 to determine just what drug residues, if any, were present in my body. I expected to find residues of the drug Ecstasy in my body as I had ingested small amounts over a period of a year or so. Needless to say, nothing could prepare me for what I was about to find. Just about every drug listed was in my body. I was amazed at the types and quantities of drugs I eventually identified. As the list got longer and longer, I remembered my experience in Maui. No wonder I had the body of a drug addict! I had acquired the drugs in a blood transfusion, and had taken on all the symptoms. This had to be very contaminated blood. Slowly, I was finding the answers I had set out to find. Piece by piece the puzzle was falling into place.

I added the list of drug residues to the long lists of other toxic substances I had identified in my body. This included organophosphate pesticides, herbicides, chemical solvents (including those uniquely military), plutonium and other types of radiation. This list was quite long by now, but it felt complete. I started the very time-consuming process of eliminating the long lists of toxic chemicals, including the drugs, from my subtle bodies with the SE5. This took months to accomplish as I had to identify and address each substance individually. Typically, it took 10-14 days to eliminate each toxin. Even at that, I found out later, I did not release the chemical residues from the cells themselves. I am still in that process, now using the blue-green algae to release and clear the individual cells.

AURA PHOTOS

As luck would have it, I had an aura photo taken with a Kirlian camera just before I began the long process of cleaning chemicals and drugs out of my body. I had never had an aura photo taken before. I took one look at the picture (figure 1) and was very disturbed by what I saw. It was very obvious that I had major holes in my aura. I had been told by psychics that drugs would create holes in the aura. I had very limited experiences with drugs. Certainly the small amounts of Ecstasy I had taken could not account for what I was seeing.

After three months of constant work with the SE5 to eliminate residues of the long lists of toxic substances from my body and brain, I had the occasion to have another aura photo taken. I was amazed and impressed with the difference in the photograph (figure 2). I noticed that the holes in the aura were now filled in, and that the vacant area around my head was now filled with color and light. I was encouraged. I was on the right track. The elimination of these toxic substances with the SE5 had produced major changes in my aura! Steadily, my energy level and mental abilities were improving.

The third picture in the series (figure 3) was taken exactly one year after the first, October 1993. I had been taking blue-green algae for two months now. (For more information on Blue-Green Algae see page 139.) Notice how much bigger and fuller the aura is. The color of my aura had also changed color from green-blue to orange and a golden yellow. This indicated that my lower chakras were opening: that residues of chemicals in the endo-crine system were being eliminated, allowing the chakras to open.

INSERT AURA PICTURES

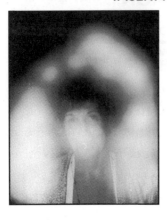

FIGURE 1: Before Clearing Drugs & Toxic Chemicals

Notice thinning and holes on left side of head and over top of head
(Color: green)

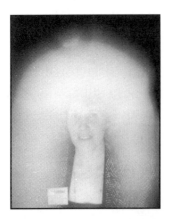

FIGURE 2: Three Months Later—Clearing Drugss & Chemicals with SE5

Aura fuller and holes filled in
(Color: green)

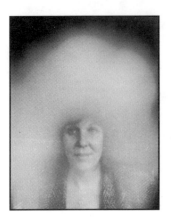

FIGURE 3: Three Months on Super Blue Green Algae™

Aura is fuller, more expanded, thicker and has changed colors
(Colors: yellow, orange, gold and red)

CONCLUSION:

The "Overgrowth" Involved With CFIDS Was Growing On Toxic Chemical Residues

Once I completed the task of eliminating the long list of toxic chemical residues from my body, I proceeded to eliminate the "overgrowth" that I had earlier identified. This included long lists of viruses, bacteria, funguses and parasites. Then, I held my breath and waited to see if the viruses would grow back. I waited. And waited. Finally, after three months, I felt confident that my theory was correct; that the viruses, funguses, bacteria, and parasites experienced by CFIDS sufferers do not grow back if the toxic substances are identified and eliminated from their subtle bodies first. Yes, I was excited! I had the information that I needed and the means to recover my health. Even today, I find that keeping the toxic chemicals eliminated from my subtle bodies will prevent the overgrowth from returning. I have not been bothered by this condition since this discovery several years ago, and my health has steadily returned.

The scientific community has spent many years researching the elusive virus. It is time to understand that viruses grow off of toxic chemicals and radioactive substances. In my reading about viruses, I remember that the first virus was identified by a man on a potato. Today, I would suspect this was a result of chemical fertilizers and pesticides on the potato.

PART 3

Sources of

Contamination

PART 3

SOURCES OF CONTAMINATION

The truth is that we are living in a very polluted world. Millions and millions of tons of toxic substances are manufactured every year. Few nations have been responsible in disposing of these chemicals. We have run out of places to dispose of them safely. Most toxic chemicals take 20-30 years to break down. Radioactive substances may take up to 24,000 years. Toxic substances are everywhere: in the air we breathe, the water and food.

Pointing the finger of blame at someone will not solve the problem. We all have to take responsibility for the world we have created to live in. We see all around us, the tangible results of the war mentality and materialistic philosophy that has been the basis of our thinking process. We have chosen to live in fear. We may be destroyed and eliminated by the very weapons and chemicals we have designed to destroy others. Unfortunately, it is not a quick death, but a very slow, painful process which will give us all a chance to understand what we have done here. Perhaps in our next incarnation, we will have learned the lesson. A higher consciousness must be presented. We are all citizens of the earth. We must be concerned for the well being of all. What touches our neighbor, also touches us. If we contaminate and pollute our earth, we will die along with her.

The earth has become a massive garbage dump. Toxic

substances, radioactive wastes and poisons are oozing out of every vein, pore and artery. She is choking and gasping for breath. We alone are responsible. We have created the garbage that now threatens to annihilate all inhabitants on earth.

FOODS IMPORTED FROM THIRD WORLD COUNTRIES

One major source of contamination is from organophosphate pesticides on food products grown in third world countries. This includes drugs, coffees, tea, cocoa, sugar, grains, herbs, fruits, and vegetables. Chances are very good that these food items contain residues of organophosphate pesticides which can be quite lethal.

As mentioned earlier, organophosphate pesticides are produced from nerve gas chemicals which are so lethal that drops can kill. Although banned in the U.S., chemical companies in the U.S. produce the pesticides and export millions of tons to third world countries. Then the food products are imported back into this country. Makes a lot of sense doesn't it?

It also seems important to mention that most drugs are grown in third world countries. Growing and exporting drugs is big business in many South American and Asian countries. Pesticides help produce bigger crops. My research has indicated a cause of concern here as well. We need to ensure that plants used in prescription durgs are free of pesticides and chemicals.

Let's face it, all pesticides are potentially lethal. Anything that is strong enough to kill bugs and pests, can also kill humans if taken in large enough quantities. Since residues of these substances remain in the body after the food is digested, if these residues build to high enough levels, there could be serious consequences to the human body.

Many third world countries have become, what I call "dumping grounds" for industrial and radioactive wastes. Newspaper articles indicate that Industrialized nations have dumped tons of radioactive wastes in Somalia. Economically impoverished governments of these small African countries have made their soils available in return for dollars. Perhaps this is why AIDS is so prevalent in Africa today.

Many third world countries have experienced wars on their soils, or have been locations of major military bases. This adds to the contamination of water and soils. They are not alone. Our waters and soils are just as polluted.

CONTAMINATED WATER SUPPLIES

Most water districts have not explored the possibility that whole arsenals of lethal chemicals might be found in the water supply, including radioactive wastes. Testing for toxic substances is quite limited. It is time to wake up to the possibility that there might be all kinds of lethal substances in the drinking water.

One must not over look the role of the military. Anyone living close to a military base is at great risk of being exposed to very lethal poisons that may have found their way into the drinking water. The possibility exists that the government has buried toxic nuclear wastes at any number of undisclosed sites. This includes toxins that could lead to the eventual development of CFIDS, or other immune dysfunction disease.

One must also be aware of places where industrial wastes have been buried in the soils, or dumped into the water. Over time, these toxic wastes will leach into the water supplies of cities and towns. Garbage dumps and toxic waste sites also pose a huge concern. For years, toxic chemicals were routinely dumped in these sites. Today, many are leaking into ground water and wells.

One must also consider the possibility of nuclear fall-out contamination from secret nuclear testing. Nuclear testing under this program continued until 1990. Fallout could affect cattle and produce farms as well as people, water and soil.

ANIMAL PRODUCTS

The animals are sick, too. Animals are contaminated by the same source as humans, primarily water and food. Toxic pesticides and chemicals will build up in the animal fat and tissues causing viruses and bacteria to grow just as in humans. There have been instances in the newspapers recently of people dying from E-Coli bacteria in contaminated beef, and articles about salmonella in chicken and chicken eggs. Another factor to consider is the large amount of antibiotics fed to the cattle. This has led to the appearance of new strains of antibiotic-resistant bacteria.

<u>Washington, DC, 1990</u>. Scientists from the Department of Agriculture found that a virus similar in genetic structure to the AIDS virus is more common in cattle in the U.S. than researchers had anticipated. The virus, bovine immunodeficiency-like virus, or BIV, is spread through the blood and is a member of a family of slow-acting viruses that have been shown to affect the immune system.

The article goes on to assure the public that this is not the AIDS virus, that we do not have the AIDS virus in cattle. However, it does say that dairy and cattle producers lose hundreds of millions of dollars each year because sick animals must be culled from their herds. They spend $300-500 million for anti-bacterial agents, antibiotics and other drugs to treat sick animals. [46]

I wonder why there are so many sick animals? If my research is correct, that the family of viruses that causes leukemia and AIDS actually grows off of radioactive waste and extremely toxic chemical solvents and pesticides, where is the source of contamination? Is this the same type of cancer-causing virus that the deer are also dying of? Could the cattle have been exposed to radioactive fallout or toxic nuclear waste dump sites from government sources? Or, is the source from pesticides? Could it be that there are several million, or more, cattle sick with CFIDS and AIDS symptoms as well as humans?

My personal research indicates that viruses, bacteria, funguses, and parasites grow off chemical pesticides, toxic solvents and radiation that build up in the tissues and organs of the animal and are eventually stored in the animal fat. Have you ever wondered how many tons of feed a steer or cow ingests in its lifetime? I bet it is a lot.

In my research, I have come across information that claims that cattle blood is so similar to human blood that, in an emergency, it could be substituted for human blood.[47] If this is true, then we are all at risk of catching any virus, bacteria or disease that cattle have. Yet, the government keeps assuring us that there is no danger. Can you really believe this?

I have found subtle energy indications of HTLV viruses in milk, cheese, and other milk products, as well as steak and other meat products right out of the grocery counter. It takes only one nice, juicy, rare steak from an infected beef to cause a lot of pain and suffering, perhaps even death. It is my personal belief that you could get any bacteria or virus, including AIDS, from infected cattle. A homeopathic practitioner in Alaska seriously believed that herpes infections were coming from cattle, as he always found certain cattle viruses, including anthrax, along with the herpes virus in clients.

It is very common for family pets to develop symptoms of CFIDS right along with the human members of the family. Everything that I just mentioned above would also apply to all family pets. In this case, I look for a common source of contamination. I would first look for toxic chemicals in the food or water, although it is possible that a virus could be transferred as well.

DRUGS

Many of the people experiencing CFIDS symptoms in Maui had a background of drug usage. Most of the drug history went back to the sixties. Some people had more recent experiences with drugs.

One of the things that became very apparent in my research was that those people with a history of drug usage in their background seemed to have heavy residues of toxic military solvents, herbicides and high levels of radiation in their subtle bodies. Today, in light of recent DOE announcements, I would suspect that the drugs have been contaminated with nuclear waste. I have to say "suspect", as I have not actually been able to analyze the drugs themselves, as possession of drugs is illegal. I have only been able to notice that certain types of toxic substances are consistently found in drug users.

I was vaguely aware of a government program that involved spraying pesticides or other chemicals on marijuana plants to eradicate them from the air. Since I did not use drugs, I did not pay too much attention to this fact. However, in my work-ups and analyses on clients experiencing CFIDS with a history of drug usage, I was finding indications of substances including: Agent Orange, organophosphate pesticides, toxic red water, lethal solvents and plutonium. I was very alarmed. The information I had on these chemicals indicated that they were extremely lethal. How could it be that they had gotten into humans in such large amounts? Was there a connection to these toxic solvents and the drugs? The more I worked, the more I believed this to be true. However, I am finding that the sources of contamination need not be from present life. Toxins from ancestors or genetic influences also seem to accumulate and can add to the problem.

I no longer work with clients who are still taking drugs, although I did when I was doing my initial research on Maui. I have learned that the energies associated with the drugs, including spirit forms on other dimensions as well as viruses, are very dangerous to deal with. Today, I will only agree to work with clients on a case by case basis. At least one year of detoxification and therapy is part of my requirement.

I have, on several occasions, had the opportunity to work with several clients with diagnosed AIDS. Again, I found the presence of large quantities of similar contaminants, including high levels of plutonium.

I have recently read that up to 50% of all AIDS patients have a background of serious drug abuse. And, since I developed HTLV 1 & 2 viruses which are in the AIDS family, I consider CFIDS a cousin to AIDS. The same information also applies to AIDS. I personally feel that AIDS, leukemia, cancer and CFIDS are all the same disease based on the same underlying cause. The determining factor as to which disease you might develop has to do with the types of chemicals you ingest, the amount of chemicals you ingest, how your liver actually breaks these chemicals down as they are digested in the body, and the history of your life experiences and those of your ancestors. In my research with people, I have discovered that people who are more likely to develop AIDS have come from different root races than people who might have predisposition to develop CFIDS. In other words, they have different experiences in their past history and have come from different genetic groups.

Intravenous drug users run a risk of getting AIDS not only from the contamination of needles by the virus, but also from the types of toxins that contaminate the drugs themselves. I personally feel that all habitual drug users will develop AIDS if they use the drugs long enough. It is simply a matter of how much lethal toxins the cells of the body can hold before they start developing viruses and disintegrating. I had an AIDS client, under hypnosis, describe the conditions involved with AIDS, as a rotting of the flesh. That feels like a pretty accurate description.

I do not wish to speculate on just how these toxic chemicals are finding their way into the drugs. However, I will state that this poses a danger to all humans. Since some prescription drugs are contaminated as well, all citizens are in danger of developing serious side effects.

BLOOD TRANSFUSIONS

We also need to look at the dangers of contaminated blood. I can speak from my own experience. I have personally lived through the hell of being given contaminated blood from a drug addict, and have taken on, not only the associated disease, but also the psychological and personality changes associated with the drugs. How many other innocent people have been put through a similar hell? How many have survived to tell their stories? Anyone taking prescription, or "over the counter" drugs, or getting a blood transfusion faces the same risk. I think the odds might be slightly better in Russian Roulette.

Looking for HIV viruses in contaminated blood is not enough. One must look for all the HTLV viruses. There is no question that these viruses are deadly and can be transmitted. However, the problem is much larger than that. One must also test for certain toxic chemicals and radiation that these viruses actually grow off. I believe that all HTLV contaminated blood may also be contaminated with plutonium, other caustic solvents, nerve gas chemicals, and other forms of nuclear waste. Even though the viruses may not be present at the time of the blood transfusion, it is possible that they will manifest at a later time. If the underlying toxic environment is present in the blood, it is only a matter of time before the viruses, bacteria, funguses, or parasites could develop. Remember that viruses are just one of the many opportunistic organisms that plutonium radiation, solvents and other toxic chemicals will spawn.

I am a stubborn person. I refused to give up the fight. Because of that, I am here today to tell you about my experience. It is not a pretty story. Many others have not, and will not, live to tell their stories. It is a story of long-term human suffering and despair. I am well today and getting stronger day by day. My body is somewhat overweight and out of shape from the years of cellular damage and inactivity. Just give me time. I will bring that back as well. I can retrace my steps for you. I have other clients who are recovering from this syndrome because of what I have shared with them. I know I am right. I know what I do works. I am here to help those who are serious about helping others through this injustice—millions of innocent people who have been and will be affected by the decisions of a powerful few who feel that war is more important than human life. We need to take a long hard look at the state of the earth and the world that we live in. We are all dying. We are not alone. Millions more will be joining the ranks of CFIDS and other immune dysfunction diseases.

PRESCRIPTION DRUGS
ARE NOT SAFE

Since my initial discovery several years ago, I have had the opportunity to analyze with the SE5, some prescription drugs which have been brought to me by clients.

I was pretty amazed and shocked at just how many times I have found the presence of residues of the same toxic solvents, pesticides and/or radiation in legal prescription drugs brought to me by CFIDS clients. Some of the drugs are solvent free, others are amazingly contaminated. Some of my clients have reported developing CFIDS symptoms after taking certain prescription drugs for an extended period of time.

A limited check in the drug store has resulted in similar discoveries concerning "over-the-counter" drugs. Analysis with the SE5 has indicated the presence of residues of toxic chemicals in some of these "over-the-counter" drugs.

I can only speculate as to why these drugs are so contaminated: 1) manufacturers of prescription drugs purchase the contaminated products from the same major suppliers-growers as the street drugs; therefore the drugs are contaminated when purchased. 2) The manufacturing plants are located near a source of major contamination, and manufacturers do not purify the water used during the manufacturing process.

WINE

Napa Valley, one of the major wine producing areas of the country, is experiencing serious problems with certain types of funguses and organisms killing off the grapes. Many vintners have been forced out of business, as their crops are being destroyed.

The same source that would result in viruses and funguses growing in the human body would also be the cause of viruses and funguses growing and destroying other living organisms, including grapevines. If this source involves nuclear waste, or radioactive fallout, then wine from other major wine-producing countries would be suspect as well. Much of Europe was contaminated with the Chernobyl explosion. There may be exposure from other nuclear testing as well.

Again, the question arises about the connection here between the grapes dying off and the deer dying off in the same area of Northern California. My mind would want to look at the possibility of radioactive fallout in this area from nuclear testing.

My discovery concerning wine was a very painful experience. I was shopping at the grocery store one day for a bottle of Champagne as a birthday gift for a good friend. After searching over the many choices of Champagne, I carefully selected a California brand in the medium price range, and placed it in the top section of the grocery cart. I proceeded a short distance, when the bottle suddenly and unexplainedly fell out of the cart and on to the top of my foot. As I saw it falling, I was paralyzed for an instant, afraid that I would be severely cut by exploding glass. My first reaction was relief, when it landed on my left foot instead of the floor. My second reaction was one of extreme pain. My foot was swollen and black and blue for several weeks.

I wondered if there was a message for me in this experience. I went back to the store and purchased a similar bottle of the same brand and proceeded to analyze it for toxic solvents and pesticides. I was once again, surprised and alarmed at the contamination I found in the wine. Purchasing other types of wine, I discovered that some brands contained similar contamination.

I feel that I need to remind you that I am talking about subtle residues of toxic substances so small that they may not show up in a typical chemical analysis. It is possible, however, that residues could be high enough to show up in a test as well. I have not had the personal finances to undertake the laboratory testing. It is important to remember that residues can accumulate and will build up in the cells and tissues of the body. Over a period of months or years, residues may reach high enough levels to cause cancer or CFIDS symptoms. Some of these substances are so toxic it does not take much to cause major problems.

PART 4

Help If You Suffer From

Chronic Fatigue Syndrome

PART 4

HELP IF YOU SUFFER FROM CFIDS

Chronic Fatigue Syndrome is truly a holistic disease. Healing must be approached from many different levels. One cannot just focus on the physical body.

DEALING WITH THE SPIRITUAL NATURE

The first area of attention is dealing with the "spiritual" aspect. If you suffer from an immune dysfunction disorder, it is important to take an honest look at your lifestyle, and "clean up your act", so to speak. You must take the first step to help yourself move into higher consciousness.

Take an honest look at the places where you are stuck and your life is not working for you. If you are addicted to drugs, alcohol, sex, or abusive relationships, you must take the first step to help yourself. Take an honest look at yourself and your life. Get involved in a therapy class, Alcoholics Anonymous, a support group, or counseling at your local church. Make sure you take the time to work with someone that you feel good about. You must care enough about yourself to make a change in your life.

I have found in my experience with clients that it does not work for me to assist people who are still involved with addictive behavior. The clearings that I do will not really hold as people will tend to draw negative influences directly back into their lives.

So, the **first step is: you must love yourself enough to want to change and to get help**.

DEALING WITH THE PHYSICAL BODY

Next, you must look at what you can do to assist your physical body.

The second step is: CHECK YOUR ENVIRONMENT FOR SOURCES OF TOXIC CHEMICALS AND RADIATION.

I. YOU MUST PURIFY YOUR WATER.

There are inexpensive water purifiers available that fit on your tap. Reverse osmosis process is the most expensive, but the best. If you can't afford this type of filter, there are some very good carbon filters. Many are multi-level marketed. Do some investigating. Read the standards. Buy the best one that you can afford.

You can buy purified water through water purifying companies. They will deliver it to your door on a regular basis. Or you can buy it in the grocery store. Be careful about buying spring water, unless you know for sure that the water source is not contaminated.

It is naive to think that because water comes out of your tap, it is safe to drink. Water companies only test for certain kinds of contaminants. This is a small and very limited list.

If you live close to a military base, or industrial area, it is even more important that you filter your water. Be very careful about drinking water at local restaurants and other places where the water is not filtered.

Also, you should realize that purifying water also takes out the minerals. So you will need to take some kind of vitamin and mineral supplements that replace them in the body.

2. EAT ORGANIC FOOD

I know it is expensive, but worth it, if you can afford to buy it. Rule of thumb is to buy organic first. If that is not possible or feasible, then buy food grown in U.S. All food is suspect.

The recent disclosures concerning our government's secret nuclear tests bring real concern about radiation pollution from radioactive fallout. Plutonium as well as pesticide residues of all kinds can be toxic. Food grown by organic means could still be contaminated by radiation.

Food additives are also chemical compounds that leave residues. It is better not to put chemicals of any kind in your body, if you can avoid it. Given the fact that chemicals are added to just about everything we put in our mouths, this is not an easy task. Do the best you can with the resources you have at hand. Since it is the nature of humans to need food and water to live, your task is to eat and drink the foods with the least possible con-tamination. Think PURE FOOD. Strive to keep what you put in your body as pure as you can.

Be very careful not to purchase food items grown in third world countries. This includes Mexico as well as Asian and South American countries.

Exercise caution when eating rice and other grains in ethnic restaurants. Find out whether they use products from U.S. or import them from their native country. Sus-pect all rice and grains.

3. WATCH YOUR DIET

You must eliminate all sweets, including sugar, honey, and fruit juices from your diet if you are plagued with chronic systemic infections. This includes systemic can-dida or other fungus as well as staph or strep infections. You might also need to eliminate bread, milk products, foods containing yeast, and most meat from your diet. Bacteria, viruses, and funguses are yeast-like in nature and feed on sugar and other sweets. Digestive distur-bances, like producing a lot of gas after eating any of the above foods may be a sign of a systemic candida in the intestinal track. If you are plagued with constant infec-tions, this may be a sign of systemic staph or strep. It is absolutely necessary to eliminate these foods from your diet if you wish to control this "overgrowth".

Meat will contain pesticide, antibiotic residues and quite possibly viruses and funguses that the animal has produced. Definitely eliminate meat that contains large amounts of fat, as chemical residues are stored in the animal fat. This would include bacon, sausage, and ham. All meat should be well cooked. Suspect eggs and chickens. There are some eggs available today that are laid by chickens fed special pesticide free diets. They are available in most stores. Look for those. Some health food stores carry meat from specially fed cattle and chickens with no pesticides or drugs. Since milk products and most beef, turkey, and chicken are also suspect, the less in your diet, the better. EAT SMALL AMOUNTS OF LEAN PROTEIN.

If at all possible, eliminate canned foods because of the food additives. Eat fresh fruits and vegetables. Food is better for you when it is raw because it contains enzymes that are often destroyed in the cooking. If you can not digest raw food, you might lightly steam your vegetables. Crisp ones still contain enzymes, so don't overcook them. Most vegetables are alkaline and will help balance the acid condition in the body. It is important to eat alkaline foods.

Investigate Ayurvedic diets. Many people have found these diets helpful in controlling CFIDS symptoms. Based on principles of ancient Indian Ayurvedic medicine, these systems determine your body type and how your body metabolizes food.

4. TAKE DIGESTIVE ENZYMES WITH EVERY MEAL.

Digestive enzymes will help you digest the food that you are eating. Remember to take a full spectrum enzyme every time you eat. Food enzymes are available in the health food stores, or can be ordered through network marketing outlets. Be careful to avoid ones that contain oxbile and other cattle products.

5. NUTRITIONAL SUPPLEMENTS/HERBS

Another very important area is nutritional supplements. Most CFIDS sufferers are deficient in magnesium and other important minerals. Many products available in the health food stores are contaminated with organophosphate pesticides because ingredients are grown in third world countries. Read the labels. Even then, there is no guarantee that products are not contaminated by radiation or other chemicals in the water supply, or other sources. Avoid supplements with yeast added, as yeast will feed the candida causing bloating and gas. Also, avoid products that contain cattle supplements like oxbile.

There are natural herbs that will kill off the "overgrowth" including bacteria causing infections, candida, ergot, parasites. There are books available on natural herbs and herbal teas, or check with your health food store for advice. Try to purchase herbs that are grown in USA.

Unfortunately, many of the really effective herbs available in the health food stores are being removed from the shelves by the Food and Drug Administration. It seems to me that there is some kind of conspiracy by the pharmaceutical companies and medical field to keep inexpensive but effective herbs out of the hands of the general public. Drugs are a big business involving millions of dollars. As many natural herbs are proven effective, they are being placed in the category of prescription drugs.

This requires that additional money be spent on doctors to obtain prescriptions. Also, I am sure we will find the price of the drugs will be many times as high as the cost in the health food stores. People, we need to get really angry and stop this practice.

Products that I have found effective for controlling candida include Capristatin and Caprisin. Capristatin is manufactured by Ecological Formulas and controls candida in the small and large intestine. Besides tablets that can be taken internally for candida, there is Orithrush Mouthwash to handle thrush (Candida in mouth and tongue) and Orithrush Vaginal Douche Concentrate, a douche for vaginal candida. These products are available in most health food stores.

Find a nutritional consultant or therapist who can use kinesiology or muscle testing to help determine your needs. Or, have a hair analysis done to determine deficiencies. I can do a pretty complete analysis on the SE5 with a sample of your hair.

6. SUPER BLUE-GREEN ALGAE™

I wish that I had discovered this product years ago. Other than the sound equipment, it is the only thing that I have found that appears to break down the crystallization of toxic chemical residues. This brand of blue-green algae seems to liquefy this chemical residue, allowing it to be eliminated from the body. Those with clairvoyant vision will see a white sticky substance coming out of the body.

If you have limited financial resources and cannot afford to do anything else, this is the place to start. This brand of blue-green algae is harvested wild from Klamath Lake, Oregon. Carefully processed, the algae is freeze dried with special equipment to retain the life force energy of this fragile substance. Super Blue-Green Algae™ is network marketed and is not available on the general retail market. Other products that I have tried to date, have not produced the same results. This includes certain types of chlorophyll, spirulina, and chlorella. Although, I am sure that they are of some benefit to ones overall health, other chlorophyll products tested do not seem to break down the chemical residues that I feel are the underlying cause of the "overgrowth" experienced by CFIDS victims. There may be other brands on the market that will do this, but I have not found them yet.

Algae is the very basis of the food chain and responsible for renewing and creating all life on this planet. Organic Super Blue-Green Algae™, or Aphanezomenon flos-aquae, is a nutrient-dense source of food. It contains all essential amino acids in near perfect ratios, vitamins, minerals, trace minerals, and neuropeptides plus more protein and chlorophyll than any other food available.

Chlorophyll is the blood of life of the plant world, and is very similar to human blood. Chlorophyll purifies the blood and oxygenates the brain, enhancing the electrical impulses in the nervous system. The chlorophyll and minerals in the algae tend to stabilize the electrons in the cells, balancing the polarity of the magnetic fields, as we talked about earlier.

Remember that toxic chemicals and elements spin in

a counter-clockwise direction. When this happens, the electrons become unstable and spin erratically. They begin shooting off in all directions. As a result of this erratic electron, the cells begin to break down. Eventually, the electrical impulses in the nervous system and brain become erratic. The thought processes and emotions may also become erratic. (This process produces free-radicals associated with aging and dis-ease.)

I feel that special ingredients in the blue-green algae work to reverse the magnetic fields of these toxic substances in the body and bring them back to a clockwise spin, creating stability within the cells. This is the spin of the "life force" of "love" energy that supports human life. Although I am not sure what ingredients in the algae allow it to do this, I suspect that it is the presence of natural cobalt combined with the DNA/RNA that is 3 1/2 billion years old that could produce this kind of electronic ancient signature. Indications are that Super Blue-Green Algae™ has not mutated throughout eons of time. A fact that may allow the energetics of this edible algae to help restore the natural rhythm and health of our cellular structure. Over time, peace, harmony and health may be restored to the cells, organs, and systems of the body as the electrons stabilize. This balance and harmony can be felt in all levels of the body.

I will say once again, I do not know of any other product on the market that will produce this result. Also, I have checked this brand of algae out for the presence of pesticides and other toxic chemical residues and the tests so far have indicated it is radiation and pesticide free.

There are several types of algae and complementary products available in this line of products which support the detoxification process of the body. It is important to start out very slowly with the algae. Detoxifying too fast will often result in symptoms of an infection or other uncomfortable symptoms, as the algae will dump viruses, bacteria and funguses into the bloodstream as it works. People with systemic infections may need to clear with infection homeopathics before they can start the algae. It is important to allow the oxygen in the algae to eliminate the organisms as they are being released. START SLOWLY AND BUILD UP.

Since there are several types of products available, it is important to find out which one your body wants to start with. I always use the SE5 to determine the type of algae to start and ideal dosage. You could use a pendulum, or kinesiology, to determine the most appropriate type of algae and the amount. Or, send me a hair sample and I can determine this for you. How long you need to take it varies again with how toxic your system is and how much damage has been done. Six months to a year is not an unreasonable length of time. Most clients begin to experience increased energy and a lessening of the symptoms in 2-3 months. These clients are working with releasing their emotional bodies along with taking the algae. Since algae is a natural food, most people will continue to take the algae as a life long program.

Besides the algae itself, there are other products available that can be taken together to produce a synergistic effect. The first one is digestive enzymes. Full spectrum enzymes are special in that they contain 20% algae in their formulation. The addition of algae to the enzymes help eliminate toxic chemicals when they are ingested with the food intake. So, pesticides and other toxic chemicals can be broken down during the digestion process and not overload the liver and other organs.

Other products that work together in this series are Acidophilus and Bifidus. Lactobacillus acidophilus is a friendly strain of bacteria that consumes sugars in the intestinal tract and produces lactic acid. It is generally found in the small intestine and enhances the digestion of food. It is very sensitive to pollutants, and is killed off by the toxin and pollutants we ingest with our food on a daily basis. Therefore, it needs to be continually reseeded in our bodies. Bifidobacterium is a beneficial intestinal bacteria that prefers to live in the colon. Both of these bacteria help to maintain optimum health. Therefore, a daily dose is recommended as well.[48]

This is a type of food. Some people may not be able to tolerate it for some reason. Be careful to start slowly and monitor your reaction to it, and act accordingly. Although I have not, personally, found anyone who was allergic to the algae, I have found taking too much will result in detoxifying too fast, sometimes resulting in an infection, excess gas, tiredness, fatigue, or sleepiness. Don't be in a hurry.

Since this product is network marketed, the only way that you can purchase it is through a distributor. I have listed a phone number and an order form in the back of this book. If you want more information on Super Blue-

Green Algae™, or wish to order products, please call me. I would appreciate your support.

Also, remember that I said that this is the place to start. Perhaps you might be one of the lucky ones who will find that this is all that is needed to regain their health. Most people, however, will need to do more. In my research, I find that it is also necessary to release the emotional body of past hurts and pains. The thymus gland which regulates the immune system is located in the heart chakra. I tell clients that healing the immune system is about healing the heart and the emotional body. The clients that I work with who get better, do both. They take the algae regularly and work with me to clear the emotional body. SO THIS IS JUST ONE OF THE STOPS FOR MOST PEOPLE. IT IS A GOOD PLACE TO START. RE-MEMBER THAT SUPER BLUE GREEN ALGAE™ IS A FOOD, NOT A MEDICINE AND THAT NO MEDICAL CLAIMS CAN BE MADE FOR ITS EFFECTIVENESS. USE YOUR GOOD JUDGMENT AND BE SURE TO CHECK WITH YOUR DOCTOR.

7. COENZYME Q-10

Investigate Coenzyme Q-10 and think about adding it to your diet. Research indicates that CoQ-10 affects the energy of the cell and is found in all cells of the body. It resembles the structure of Vitamin K and is considered essential for the health of all the cells, tissues and organs of the body. Studies have recently linked the absence of this enzyme with the aging process of cells. Deficiencies of this enzyme can result in medical conditions including cardiovascular disease, heart failure, and hypertension. It has been found to be an important element in longevity and appears to counteract side effects of prescriptions drugs, is effective in treating periodontal disease, diabetes mellitus and obesity, and in strengthening the immune system.[49]

8. HOMEOPATHIC REMEDIES

Investigate the use of homeopathic remedies to assist you in eliminating such things as food poisoning (very common in CFIDS because of not digesting food), systemic staph and strep infections, systemic candida and viruses that you may have in your body. You might also be able to clean out radiation and toxic pesticides from your system as well.

You will probably need to take the remedies for a longer time than usual because of a weak immune system. Remember to mention this to the practitioner. Keep in mind that they will grow back in a matter of weeks or months.

However, you will find the increase in energy worth the money. Eliminating this overgrowth that is draining the energy of the body will improve your energy level and outlook on life. It will buy you some valuable time, if you can afford it.

9. DETOXIFICATION

Begin a detoxification program. There are many available. Blue-Green Algae will detoxify your system. If you have been exposed to radiation or have taken drugs there may be some very specific detox programs for you. Besides taking algae, consider adding colon cleansers to your daily routine. They will begin the process of cleaning out mucus and toxic build-up in the colon which is a breeding ground for fungus, bacteria, and parasites.

Investigate having a colonic. These are often unpleasant experiences, but you would be surprised at the debris that builds up in the intestines during years of digestion. It is well worth it to have this done at least once in your life. You will be eliminating the habitat of many organisms that do not promote a healthy body. Be sure to check with your doctor for his advice.

10. SOUND

As I have mentioned earlier, sound can be an effective tool to identify and eliminate toxic substances from your body and energy field. It can also be used to clean out and eliminate pesticides and chemical fertilizers from your food before you eat it.

The SE5 is available for purchase at $2500. It will speed up the process of eliminating the residues of toxic chemicals and is a very valuable tool to have if you can afford one. I have lists available of the toxic pesticides and chemicals I have identified to date. The SE5 can be used to effectively eliminate these substances from the energy bodies. It is very helpful in removing contaminating chemicals from food, drink, and supplements before they are ingested. Just about everything is contaminated on some level. So, I highly recommend looking into one. It could be a valuable aid to your recovery process. I personally feel that I owe my life to it.

11. REIKI

Reiki is an ancient tradition using life force energy channeled through the hands of a trained practitioner to release blockages from the subtle bodies. Many Reiki practitioners are also clairvoyant which allows them to "see" energy blockages on other dimensions.

Investigate having a Reiki session, then evaluate how you feel afterwards. Look for a practitioner who is clairvoyant and can tell you whether you have this white cement-like chemical residue buildup in your brain. Reiki can help begin the process of breaking it down. The type and quality of the energy channeled will vary with the clarity and vibrational frequency of the practitioner. Shop around. Use your intuition.

12. THERAPEUTIC MASSAGE & BODY WORK

There are many good types of energy work available which will help flush blockages and stuck energy through your body. Generally speaking, energy work such as massage will tend to work layer by layer to free this stuck energy and release it from the physical body. Once again, the clearer and higher the vibration of the therapist, the more energy will be released. Don't let people work on you who smoke, use drugs, or drink alcohol. Ask questions before you let someone touch your body. The touch itself can be very healing. Most of us have not been touched enough as children and adults. This is a very healing and therapeutic process. If you cannot afford to pay someone for a professional massage, much benefit can be derived from a loving massage from a mate or partner. There are instructional videos available on massage techniques.

13. INVESTIGATE AND ELIMINATE ALL TOXIC CHEMICALS FROM YOUR HOUSE

So many of the products that we find in our homes today are made from synthetic and often toxic materials. This includes carpeting, furniture, curtains, drapes, clothing, cleaning solvents, and furniture polish. Read the labels before you open the can or bottle and inhale the assortment of chemicals that might be present. A toxic body will often react adversely to exposure to other toxic substances. BE AWARE. BE PRUDENT.

14. EDUCATE YOURSELF ABOUT ELECTROMAGNETIC FIELDS AND THE DANGERS OF ELF WAVES.

A Polarizer is a complex crystal antenna system designed to neutralize and balance the harmful effects of man-made electrical and electromagnetic energies in home, office, computers, and from transmissions of TV, radio, telephone, microwave, radar and high tension power lines. The Polarizer will reverse the reverse spin of subatomic particles created by electrical and electromagnetic field pollution. It is said to neutralize the frequency wave lengths that have lost their natural resonance of vibrational spin and enhance the normal spin and amplitude strength of naturally occurring energy wave forms.

It is believed that constant exposure to counter-clockwise electromagnetic radiation from power lines and electrical wiring gradually exhausts the body's defense mechanisms weakening the immune system. This further interferes with its ability to fight off bacteria, viruses, toxin and cancer-producing agents. This seems to be the same type of effect the toxic chemicals themselves have on the body. The idea is that a sick, already toxic body, can be further weakened by the bombardment of electromagnetic radiation from just about any electrical source. This becomes extremely important if you work regularly with a computer.[50]

A small Polarizer can be purchased for $75 that will handle all appliances on the same electrical system. This is a worthwhile investment.

There are several books that talk about the dangers of ELF Waves. It may be dangerous to your health to live near radio stations, TV antennas, microwave towers, and high transmission lines. Educate yourself.

There is a form on the last page of this book which you can use to request more information on Polarizers, or to order one.

15. MAGNETS

Magnets also can be quite helpful in the case of CFIDS or other immune dysfunction disease. As mentioned before, toxic chemicals of all kinds, including radiation, have a counterclockwise spin. This spin seems to create erratic electrons that shoot off and result in the breakdown of molecules, atoms, and subatomic particles. Almost everything that is detrimental to the functions of the life force necessary for humans to thrive will have a counterclockwise spin.

Magnets are another device that can help reverse this counterclockwise spin in the body. How quickly they will help depends on how toxic the body is and the strength of the magnets as well as the length of time that you use them.[50]

You can purchase magnetic strips that can be placed under the mattress. Also, you can wear magnets taped to the body. These magnets can be purchased at an electrical supply store, or write to Edmund Scientific for a current catalog. The address is 101 E. Gloucester Pike, Barrington, New Jersey, 08007-1380. There are other magnetic products available specifically designed by professionals to help relieve common problems associated with reversed electromagnetic fields. These products are a lot more expensive. You can write or call me for more information on these magnets. AGAIN, THE FDA DOES NOT ALLOW ANY MEDICAL CLAIMS TO BE MADE ABOUT THESE PRODUCTS. YOU MUST READ THE LITERATURE AND DECIDE FOR YOURSELF AS TO ITS EFFECTIVENESS.

CLEARING THE SUBTLE BODIES

The third area you must focus your attention on is releasing the emotional body as well as the other subtle bodies. In most cases, it is not enough to just deal with the physical body. Believe it or not, I have found that in most cases, working only with the physical body will not usually relieve the symptoms of CFIDS. It seems to be equally important to clear and release the subtle bodies as well. I have begun to suspect, as a result of this work, that there is a very definite genetic factor, or predisposition.

My memories of the earth's history indicate that there were many different root races that populated the earth during millions of years. At different times, these different root races have come and gone from this planet. If what I have seen is true: that many of these root races are indeed dying races today, then we need to look at the possibility that their genes carried within humans today, are also breaking down.

Traditional thinking of the medical and scientific community will tell you that it is impossible to release this genetic predisposition; I feel strongly that this is what I am doing in my work with past life regression clearings. The more I do this work, the more convinced I become that this is possible. In order to understand just how this works, I will give you some information on the makeup of the subtle bodies that are an important part of the makeup of all humans. You cannot see them, but they are there. So let's take a look at them and how they function.

The physical body is the end result of the electrical information contained in the blueprint of the different subtle bodies. Every organ and system of the physical body has its subtle body counterpart. A clairvoyant when looking at the biofield, will see colors flashing in different shades and at different frequencies. On some level, she must understand the principles of color and sound in order to translate this coded information into words. These vibrating color and sound codes can be expressed in many ways. They are in effect a bridge between conscious and unconscious worlds, a bridge between energy, thoughts, or feelings expressing as emotions through matter.

One might think of matter as frozen color and sound frequencies organized into patterns. The color and sound patterns first organize in electromagnetic fields at the subatomic level. As this field densifies and crystallizes, it creates an electrical charge at a specific frequency. This electrical charge manifests as the various elements and provides the chemical bonding for the states of matter: gas, liquids, or solids. Energy is first electromagnetic in nature before molecular. The biofield may govern the chemical processes in humans from the cellular level, thus affecting the final outcome of the physical level. [51]

If this is true, then dysfunction and dis-ease at the physical level is a result of disorder at the subtle energy level. If we desire to make changes in the physical, it may be easier and more effective to make those changes in the subtle bodies. Because the subtle bodies are less dense than the physical, it becomes easier to make changes in the way the subatomic particles align in molecules and atoms at the physical level.

Often changes in the subtle bodies will result in changes in the physical body as well. Sometimes these changes are so subtle they will not be detected on the conscious level. Other times, these changes can be quite profound.

Eastern philosophies and metaphysical teaching tell us that the human biofield contains more than one body, each with its own specific function and coded vibrational information.

Let's take a closer look at the makeup of the body. Please refer to the diagram on page 159. You will see the location and identification of the different bodies that are involved in the makeup of humans.

THE SOUL BODY

Located at the outermost ring is the Causal or Soul Body. It is the least dense of all the bodies, vibrating at the highest frequency. The soul contains the highest component of self, or god consciousness. This is the place where all learning and information, from all incarnations, is recorded. The frequency that the soul vibrates on usually has to do with the age of the soul: older souls seem to vibrate at a higher light frequency than newer ones.

The souls that I deal with on a daily basis seem to come in all sizes and shapes: 1) they can be fused with other souls 2) fragmented 3) torn 4) come with grotesque spirit forms attached 5) and be otherwise battered and bruised. I would say that most of us are wounded soldiers, survivors of many lifetimes of trauma, and the souls that I work with very much show this in their appearance. I find very few souls that are bright reflections of light, or even symmetrical in shape for that matter. Most of us are vibrating on the third dimensional plane, and our souls reflect that.

153

As traumatic memories of lifetime experiences are healed and released, the soul vibrations will increase and will hold more light. Then it is possible to think about connecting with the higher self, or god self, again. This higher self may also be called an oversoul. Most of us are fragments of a larger oversoul. As our individual souls are cleaned and polished, and begin to hold more light, we will again connect to this oversoul. This process is known as Ascension. There is much information coming forth at this time concerning this process.

THE MENTAL BODY

The Mental Body is located adjacent to the Soul Body, the next ring in. Some people feel that this body is still evolving and is more like an ellipse in shape and does not fully surround the body like the others. For our purposes, we will assume that the mental body is the same size and shape as the other subtle bodies. The mental body is more dense than soul body, but less than the emotional body. The function of the mental body is to process thought by integrating and interpreting sensory data. Its basic color will vary with the interests of the individual. A mentally active person with much knowledge will have shades of yellow, orange, and gold present in this portion of the aura. Depression will be represented by dark, murky colors.

All the negative beliefs of our ancestors, and negative decisions based on personal experiences are recorded in this body. I strongly feel that its function is influenced by drugs and chemicals from past life experiences as well. It is not unusual to find spirit forms, or entities, attached or assigned to this body.

THE EMOTIONAL BODY

The Emotional Body, or Astral Body, is the next ring in. It is more dense than the mental body and vibrates at a slower frequency. It is the vehicle which allows us to process feelings, acting as a bridge between the mind and the physical body. Both positive and negative emotions are recorded in this body. This includes our fears, anger, resentments, pain as well as hopes and dreams. Emotions not expressed, over time, will crystallize in this body becoming dense, dark crystals which are eventually stored in the unconscious mind. These dark crystallized emotions send out a vibration which tends to attract others into our lives that hold similar vibrational patterns of emotion.

Suppose we have a habit of repressing anger for many lifetimes. Over time, the anger emotions will slow down and become stagnant, then tar-like and sticky, and finally become a dark crystalline substance. As these emotions densify, they send out a vibration that draws other angry people into our lives who will mirror our repressed anger.

This crystallization of repressed emotions is the reason that we find it very hard to break out of old patterns and ways of doing things. The crystallized energy tends to hold the pattern in place. Modern therapy tends to chip away at this crystallized energy, piece by piece. Hypnosis offers a way to release the energy much more quickly.

THE ETHERIC BODY

The Etheric Body is located adjacent to the physical body between the Emotional and the Physical Bodies. It is the most dense of the subtle bodies. As the "architectural blueprint" of the physical body, it functions to transfer life energy from the universal life force to the individual through a system of meridians, chakras and glands. This life force energy has many names, including prana and chi. At the etheric level the life force is taken in by the chakras and meridians, then transferred to the physical level via the glandular system. Little is understood about just how this works.

AKASHIC RECORDS

Every particle of physical matter has its etheric counterpart. The etheric material also contains all the lifetime experiences of the individual and his ancestors. These records are called "Akashic records" by psychics and metaphysicians. Many psychics can read these Akashic records and are able to give an individual information about past incarnations.

It has been my experience that included in these records are diseases and toxic substances experienced by the individual and his ancestors throughout lifetimes. It is my belief that this dense etheric Akashic substance is wrapped around the DNA, creating a membrane which serves as a veil that keeps us from being able to understand or connect with our "godself" or "higher self". The more unresolved traumatic lifetimes we have in our cellular memory, the thicker this membrane.

In my own healing process, I have spent years accessing and processing information from this veil. Over the years, I feel that I have relived and released over 650 traumatic lifetimes. In my case, this veil was extremely thick and dense, contributing to the very dense physical vibration. I would be considered a very ancient soul, as my origins go back very far. By peeling the onion, layer by layer, I intuitively healed lifetimes of repressed trauma and emotions. Layer by layer, the residues of these lifetimes were released from my DNA. Slowly, my energy levels increased as well as the function of my immune system and nervous system.

It is also my belief that as past life memories of traumatic experiences are remembered and healed, this Akashic membrane actually breaks off from around the DNA and can be flushed out of the body through the blood and lymph system. Massage and other types of energy work assist in the process of flushing out old influences and clearing them from the physical body. They can also be released with inaudible sound technology like the SE5, and the Blue-Green Algae, CoQ10, and other detoxifying agents.

THE BODY ACTS LIKE
A COMPUTER

To help you understand this, let's pretend that the human vehicle with all of its bodies is really a sophisticated computer system. Everything that has happened to this computer, from its inception, is recorded somewhere in this system. Let us also pretend that each lifetime that this human has experienced is recorded in its very own special software program. Information for this software program is coded in all of the subtle bodies.

Therefore, a person's emotional experiences are recorded in the emotional body, the mental beliefs and decisions are recorded in the mental body, organs and major system functions as well as malfunctions (diseases) are recorded in the etheric body, etc. The really traumatic lifetimes with unresolved emotions and issues are the real problem software programs. The happy lifetimes tend to come and go without much attention or residue, perhaps because the original computer program was built this way. However, the traumatic lifetimes leave major imprints on the original program and tend to overlay the original function of the computer. Unresolved emotional issues and negative decisions of these lifetimes tend to actually affect the overall system. Layer upon layer, lifetime upon lifetime, these effects accumulate and change how the system operates.

Today, the human body is a result of the accumula-

Your Subtle Bodies

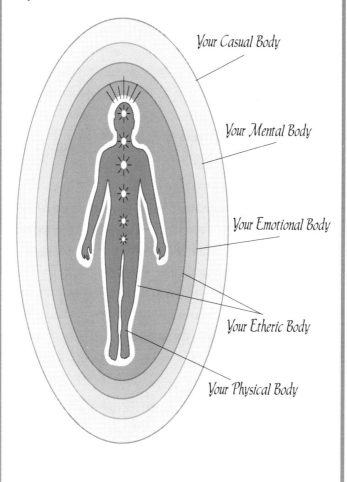

Your Casual Body

Your Mental Body

Your Emotional Body

Your Etheric Body

Your Physical Body

tion of all these software programs, and, as a result, few actually function at optimal levels. The reason why there is so much dysfunction in society at all levels is that we are walking around with all the dysfunction from hundreds of lifetimes built into the physical body. Not all of this information is our own personal experience; some of it is our ancestors, who are in our genetic lineage. Their traumatic experiences are also recorded in our computer systems.

Unresolved emotions as they densify and crystallize, are eventually stored in the hard drive memory where they are constantly being activated. These traumatic lifetime experiences tend to take up a lot of space. The computer is constantly trying to release and resolve these on its own.

Old software programs can be activated and brought into the present program in several ways. This includes meeting people who were in those lifetimes, visiting places where traumatic situations actually took place, or having similar situations occur in present life. Sometimes these old programs can be released, or worked through, by working out problems in the present life. Also, some can be released with physical activity, exercise, massage, or other types of energy work including therapy.

Most of them, however, continually back up on the other side of the physical, where they seem to have a very important effect on the function at the physical level even though they do not reside in the physical body. The negative beliefs, decisions and the unresolved crystallized emotions, combined with toxic substances and diseases experienced in each life-time, together produce a heavy vibrational weight that tends to make the physical body very dense and lock it into the third dimension. The more of these traumas that have "stacked up", the thicker the membrane or veil around the DNA, the heavier and more depressed the physical body may become. The physical body may actually become fatigued and physically ill because of this energy backing up.

Hypnosis allows a way to access these unresolved traumas and to release and heal these software programs. As one begins the process of releasing these programs, the energy lightens up and the physical body often feels better, sometimes immediately.

In the work that I have done, I find that I can often help others release these patterns very quickly. An individual will tend to create many lifetimes with the same people where very similar emotional situations are rec-reated over and over again. It is not uncommon to find that a person may have had 40-50 lifetimes where a very similar emotional trauma was created with the same people. The more lifetimes that one creates the same pattern, the harder it is to break free of the pattern in present life. In my case, I have had to relive each lifetime and release it individually.

As a result of the information that I have learned doing this work for years, I have created ways to effectively release all similar lifetimes including the people involved, as well as spirit forms that might also be involved. It is no longer necessary for clients to "peel the onion, layer by layer" for years. I have shortened this process considerably so that clients often experience relief in just a few sessions. As a result of the work, old patterns in relationships or other aspects of their lives can be released quickly and these aspects of their lives clear up almost immediately. This also works with CFIDS clients.

As I mentioned earlier, traditional counseling methods including hypnosis techniques would probably take 40-50 sessions to chip away and release these deeply ingrained patterns. Quite possibly, many sessions would be required just to get through the drama created in the present life, let alone getting to the root of the situation in past incarnations. This is truly unique work which is very effective for those who are sincerely ready to make changes in their lives.

THE HISTORY OF EVOLUTION OF HUMANS

Although many scientists will disagree with me on this, I have come to some very definite personal beliefs about the history of the earth and the people on it, based upon my personal memories of my journey here.

I strongly believe that there are several different types of humans on the planet today. Some races are evolving upward in an evolutional spiral. Some of these races indeed have their origins from primates. There were many different groups that came to earth and seeded races. Some of these races were hybrids: cross-bred from extraterrestrials with humans or primates. Other races, including the ones in which I have my origins, came into this planet as Ascended Beings or Masters of Light. Many of us, most recently, came from a star system known as the Pleiades. These light beings had the experience on Earth of spiraling downward into matter because of certain events that happened here, including the dramas that were played out, especially in Atlantis.

Millions of years ago these Beings of Light did not have physical bodies, and were much less dense in makeup. These were the gods and goddesses referred to in our mythology. Their bodies vibrated at a much higher frequency then ours today. These Light Beings were devoted to the philosophy of "service to others" and the principles of love and caring.

Atlantis began the trend toward rational thinking, and gradually things started to change. Time brought a shift from the heart-centered philosophy of love, to one of rational, left-brain intellectual thinking. As we began to perceive the world with our brains rather than our hearts, our vibrations slowed down and our bodies began to densify. At that point in time, we possessed the ability to create our world with our thoughts, and were able to manifest the results almost immediately.

Thus we began to create limitation by our negative thoughts: restricting who we were by our thoughts. Another word for this process would be limitation, or limited thinking: restricting who we are by our thoughts. We created tightness or restriction in our beings. Layer by layer, through many incarnations these restrictive thoughts densified and condensed around our soul in the form of DNA. Throughout millions of years, and thousands of incarnations, unresolved emotional traumas and negative decisions created restriction and lowered the vibrations. Today, we find ourselves trapped in these dense, vibrationally heavy bodies.

Keep in mind that the earth itself was a much lighter vibration as well. As Light Beings in the early days of earth, we did not experience death. As time went by, and the planet aged, we became more dense and started to age and experience death.

There have been many high civilizations on earth. One of those high vibrational times is known as Lemuria today. The original residents of Lemuria did not experience death. Millions of years later, at the beginning of Atlantis, the life span had shortened considerably and death was a reality for most inhabitants. As Atlantis aged the life span of its inhabitants shortened as well. So we see a gradual progression of life span downward to perhaps 150,000, then 75,000 years, and finally 2000-1500 years at the end of Atlantis. We see a similar aging process recorded in the bible as we read the old testament. Today, we are lucky to reach 90 years or so. [52]

This shortened life span was caused by the impact of the vibrational density added to the bodies by crystallized and unresolved emotions, traumas, and toxic substances. Time will show that there were many traumatic events, including nuclear wars during the time of Atlantis.

In order to release the influence of this process on our physical bodies today, it becomes necessary to relive and release the experiences. This process eventually allows us to lighten up our vibration and release the density that has locked us into the third dimensional vibration . It also allows us to heal and release genetic influences that predispose us to certain diseases from our DNA.

COMMON ENERGY DRAINS IN CFIDS CLIENTS

I find that many people who have CFIDS often share similar past life experiences which are recorded in the DNA. I will discuss those here.

LIFETIME OF REPRESSED EMOTIONS

Most CFIDS clients have habitually repressed their emotions for many lifetimes. In many cases, they no longer feel or experience their emotions. Underlying issues are involved with self-love, self-esteem and invasion of personal space. For most women, this includes lifetimes of rape and abuse. Many times clients don't know how to set boundaries or limitations. Issues arise concerning proper discernment of others.

These patterns are old and deep, and repeated in this lifetime as well. As mentioned earlier, repressing emotions such as rage and anger lifetime after lifetime will effect the personal power of an individual. This involves the third chakra where digestion and assimilation of food takes place. When these chakras are shut down, energy levels in the physical body are affected. Also, the heart chakra is usually closed and filled with grief, which affects the immune system.

The clients who experience the fastest recovery are those who are willing to work to unlock their emotions. This allows the heart to open and feelings to be experienced. Energy levels begin to rise as well.

MEMORIES OF NUCLEAR HOLOCAUST

Many, if not all, clients with CFIDS seem to have memories of nuclear holocaust or some other type of explosion in common. Information is coming to light that there have been times of major nuclear holocaust in the history of the earth. Several dates have come up consistently.

I have relived memories of a nuclear disaster around 1200 BC. In my memories of this experience, some kind of nuclear weapons arsenal was exploded in Egypt. The wind then blew this hot nuclear cloud over most of what is now the Middle East today, where it exploded another nuclear arsenal around the area of the Tigris-Euphrates and then began to backlash. The results of this disaster were experienced as far east as the Indus Valley. People were instantly incinerated. The land was parched. This land was not originally desert, but had green brush and vegetation. There was little warning and few survivors. Interestingly enough, several of my clients have relived the same memory and have even come up with the same dates. Victims were performing a variety of activities one would do in a typical day, when suddenly, out of nowhere, this black cloud appeared and all were instantly incinerated.

CFIDS clients who have this experience recorded in their DNA have also shown high subtle energy indications of radiation, including plutonium and radioactive fallout, and certain toxic chemicals in their biofield. They may also experience major energy drains because of the damage to the various bodies at the time of the nuclear experience.

The "software" program which has recorded all of this information still tells the computer that there was major dysfunction and damage to all organs and systems of the body. This software program may be activated and overlay the physical body with the old information, thereby greatly affecting the function of the present physical body. It is common in this situation to find indications of major damage to the subtle bodies as well, including the soul body.

The intensity of the nuclear blast is one of the few things that is capable of severely damaging the soul body. It can be fragmented, split, fused, or completely destroyed. It may take many lifetimes to repair the damage of a surviving soul. A soul that has been completely destroyed would be totally lost and recycled to start the process all over again. No one is immune or safe from this experience, even ancient souls are at risk of complete destruction.

Damage experienced by a surviving soul could bring

much confusion and "darkness" in subsequent incarnations because of a combination of the radiation and toxic chemicals present and the actual damage to the subtle and physical bodies. This would manifest as mental or psychological problems, or even major dis-ease in the physical body.

If you want more information about nuclear holocaust on the earth I recommend several books. The first one is by Zacharia Sitchen, entitled **The Wars Between Gods and Men.** Sitchen's books are based upon translations of ancient Akkadian and Sumerian tablets, some of the oldest records on this planet. In this book, he talks about a nuclear holocaust that happened in the Middle East. He comes up with a slightly different date from mine.[53]

Another book of interest **Viamana Aircraft of Ancient India and Atlantis,** by David Childress. This book is based upon documents which have survived from the history of ancient India that were interpreted from a language that pre-dated Sanskrit. Stories in these records talk about nuclear wars that happened about 5000 years ago. These ancient documents record wars between residents of Atlantis and residents of the continent which is called India today. The records also describe, in detail, how ships were made, how they were powered, and the nuclear and laser weapons that were in existence at that time. This is a very interesting book. [54]

Recent archaeological findings in the area of the Indus Valley indicate that something was experienced there, in the ancient past, that was hot enough to fuse the sand into green glass. Sitchen also talks about this occurring in the Sinai desert. One of the few things capable of generating enough heat to cause this type of reaction would be an atomic or nuclear explosion.

These types of explosions cause major damage to the subtle bodies. Often major parts of the soul are fragmented or destroyed. The subtle bodies experience rents, tears, and missing parts. Energy can leak from the subtle bodies because of the damage. Very often toxic chemicals and radiation from the explosion are still in the etheric substance and are either leaking into the physical, or can somehow affect its function from the etheric level.

I am not totally sure how this is done, but I do know it has a very definite effect. Horrible and frightening life forms that are born out of the explosion may be attached to the soul. Groups of people may have been fused together by the intensity of the heat. All of these things can and do contribute to the energy leakage from the subtle bodies of CFIDS clients.

DRUGS AND POISONS FROM PAST LIFE EXPERIENCES.

Another factor that seems to be at work with my CFIDS patients is the influence of toxic drugs and poisons from other lifetimes. I feel that residues of these toxins are still present in the etheric body and, again, are either leaking into the physical or can affect it from the etheric matter. The result felt in the physical body includes extreme fatigue and often symptoms of slow poisoning.

For instance, clients whose analysis with the SE5 indicates the presence of large amounts of arsenic or belladonna present in their subtle bodies, will probably remember under hypnosis lifetimes where they were poisoned, or were incarnated into societies which used these substances in rituals. Perhaps the very presence of the poison in the subtle bodies can cause these symptoms, as I am not totally sure how this works. I do know that when these lifetimes are healed and the toxin released, CFIDS clients will often experience immediate relief.

Many women who suffer symptoms of CFIDS or Chronic Fatigue may recall many lifetime incarnations where drugs or other hallucinogenic substances were routinely used on a day-to-day basis. Women often served as high priestesses or were "sacrificial virgins".

Information from clients indicates that drugs were used in spiritual rituals and practices in many different societies. As the vibrational frequencies lowered on earth, and Light Beings began to lose their superhuman, godlike, abilities to heal people and telepathically communicate with each other and with those Masters and Beings on higher planes, drugs were introduced into the temples which allowed the high priests and priestesses to "see" into other dimensions and obtain information. There seemed to be many different types of societies which encouraged the use of drugs as a spiritual experience to commune with the gods.

I was struck by a famous plaque from an ancient Greek temple, showing Demeter, the Great Mother Goddess, holding poppies in her hands. Poppies are a source of opium. Opium and drugs made from opium are just one of the many types of drugs that clients remember taking in these ancient lifetimes.

As a result of my work, I am becoming more and more aware of the role that drugs played in the downfall of these gods and goddesses. Drugs and hallucinogenic substances used in temple rituals condemned many goddesses to lifetimes in the "underworld". I also feel that drugs contributed to the violent, abusive, and warlike behavior of the gods, such as Zeus, and the wars that were waged during mythological times. Once the drugs were ingested, residues were carried over into other lifetimes, allowing the "dark forces" attached to the drugs on other planes and dimensions to influence and control the users. In other words, my work indicates that the "negative or dark forces" were attached to the chemicals in the drugs. As long as there are drugs in the body, one cannot be free of these detrimental influences on other planes. That is also the case today.

I find that residues of drugs from other life times still exist in the Akashic etheric substance around the DNA. They can very definitely contribute to the fatigue experienced with CFIDS today. These drugs need to be identified and the life-time memories released. Then they will release into the bloodstream where they can be released from the system.

Mayan and Inca rituals commonly used a drug known as datura. Also known as Torna Loco, I suspect that we will eventually find a connection to residues of this drug and mental illnesses experienced today, such as paranoia and schizophrenia. I also feel that people who are addicted to drugs today most likely have been involved with drugs in the past. It is the presence of residues of these past life drugs that keeps the addiction in place and makes it very difficult for that individual to resist drugs in the present life.

In one of my more recent experiences, I remembered being kidnapped, drugged, and raped in the area know today as England about 300 AD. I very clearly saw that the drug used at that time was cocaine. Analysis with the SE5 indicated large residues of this drug present in my subtle bodies immediately after reliving this experience.

Work with other clients have revealed very similar experiences where residues of the drug were identified in the subtle body before a hypnosis session. During that session information was obtained evolving usage of these drugs during a past life incarnation. I have devised methods to flush residues of drugs out of the subtle bodies during the hypnosis sessions. Then I find that follow-up with the Blue-Green Algae or CoQ10 will most often flush them out of the body.

I have accumulated a long list of hallucinogenic plants or mushrooms used in spiritual rituals throughout South America, Mexico, Africa, and Europe. Drugs include opium, datura, belladonna, some types of LSD, cocaine, mushrooms, cactus, and other hallucinogenic plants. It is not unusual to find residues of these drugs in CFIDS clients. Many of these clients have not had drug experiences in this lifetime.

Research seems to indicate that residues of drugs can contribute to the CFIDS symptoms experienced by these clients. Once the lifetimes are accessed and the experienced released and healed, the client will usually experience psychological and often physical relief of symptoms. This has led me to believe that residues of these substances are somehow present in the DNA of these clients, at least the vibrational frequency of the drugs or poisons are present.

I have recently come across some channeled information that validates the experience and conclusions I have come to as a result of my own research. This information is channeled by Bob Fickes, and can be found in his book entitled **Ascension, the Time is Now.**

SPIRIT FORMS OR ENTITIES

The third major source of energy drain experienced in immune dysfunction involves beings on other dimension or planes that do not have physical bodies. Sometimes these energy forms once had a physical body. The popular movie, <u>GHOST,</u> with Whoopi Goldberg did a fairly accurate job of portraying this phenomena. This type of spirit form is commonly known as a discarnate being or astral shell. A discarnate being is distinguished from another type of spirit form that has never existed in a physical incarnation. These types of spirit forms more closely resemble the energies we know as nature spirits, fairies, and angels. However, they would be a polarized opposite in vibration and design.

Discarnate Beings for various reasons do not go to the "light" after death, but choose to hang around the earth after death. Some may not believe in an afterlife. Others may stay to be with loved ones for a time. Still others are addicted to drugs, alcohol, and sex and want to continue these experiences while on the other side.

Discarnates need to attach to a human energy source to exist. Similar habits, beliefs, or emotional patterns will allow them to attach to an individual, where they can access and drain off the life force. In fact, the host individual might suddenly take up smoking, or take on suicidal thoughts, or make other major changes in his personality due to the influence of the spirit form. Sometimes, the discarnates have been attached to an individual for many lifetimes. In most cases, the host individual might have difficulty distinguishing his own thoughts from the discarnate's thoughts. Once discovered, these energy forms can be removed and released to the light.

It is not unusual for an individual to become fused with one or more discarnates because of some experience in the past. For instance, it is quite possible that beings adjacent to one another during the time of an intense explosion or holocaust might actually experience their souls being fused together because of the intense heat.

There are other reasons that might result in souls getting fused with one another. Murdering or killing someone would cause this type of fusion. People sacrificed to volcanoes will often be fused with really toxic minerals from the volcanoes. Making vows of "undying love" to another person will fuse two people together. Performing rituals of black magic will fuse people to beings on other dimensions who do their bidding.

Another type of spirit form has never lived in a human body. These types of spirits are often attached to the chemicals in plants and drugs. Just as devas and fairies are the guardians of flowers and trees, there is a polar opposite. These beings are reflected in the grotesque and demonic representations we see in symbols of the ancient past. They can represent energies that are harmful or poisonous to the human system. In most cases, there is an attempt to control the host individual in some manner. Once again, this influence can be stopped and the beings released.

Someone suffering from AIDS or CFIDS will be host to a large array of spirit forms. I routinely find 60 to 90 entities attached to these people. I have come to believe that the toxic chemicals in the body are actually breeding these "perverted", or negative life forms, and that there is a relationship between the types of entities and the types of viruses in the body. For instance, when working with someone who has manifested the HTLV 1 & 2 viruses in his body, I will always find one group of extraterrestrial entities known as Zetas working with them on some level. With HIV, there seems to be a connection with another group known as Draco beings: vampires, vampire bats, and dracula-type characters.

It is my feeling that entities have a hierarchical system of evolution just as most life forms do. Starting with a simple entity and becoming more complex as you follow the chain of command upward, I feel that this system relates directly to the growth of funguses, bacteria, mycobacteria, viruses, and finally parasites found in the human body. In fact, I feel that these are actually parasitic life forms feeding off the human host. When you actually get into the process of identifying the form attached to the specific virus, bacteria, or parasite, you get insight into the personality of the life form.

As one focuses on clearing and removing the residues of toxic chemicals and drugs from the body, many entities will also disappear. If the clearing is in this fashion, often there is no need to depossess these spirit forms, as many will disappear by themselves.

CONCLUSION

As I have stated earlier, it is my opinion, based upon my own experience with healing Chronic Fatigue Syndrome, that this is a dysfunction based on toxic chemicals, including radiation and nuclear waste. The conditions that exist today on the earth are making it very hard for all oxygen-breathing life forms to continue to exist.

After years of my own personal struggle to survive, I have made it through to the other side, and have created a path for others to follow. I have clients who are also recovering. My process includes the use of a natural food, Blue-Green Algae, CoQ10 and homeopathics to detoxify the body, and the use of hypnosis to release major traumatic experiences from the genetics of the DNA. It is quick and effective for those who are open to the process.

In truth, there is only one real cure: a higher consciousness that calls for the complete elimination of the fear-based philosophy that we have lived under for thousands of years. We have to face ourselves and the fact that we are slowly but surely killing ourselves and each other by the feeding of this fear.

We must stop the manufacture and production of toxic chemicals and the weapons of war. Most importantly, this includes nuclear warfare. We must stop the production of plutonium and the testing of nuclear bombs as well as technology that uses this nuclear power to generate energy.

We must call for the elimination of the production of nerve gas chemicals whether for war or for pesticides.

The choice is a simple one: to chose life or death. The state of this planet would indicate that all existing life forms are in the process of extinction. It is only a matter of time.

I offer a cure here. Perhaps there are others that will come to light as well, but all of this is temporary if major efforts of massive cleanup of our environment are not undertaken immediately.

We have the technology available to us. It is simply a matter of focusing this technology on the elimination of toxic chemicals rather than war.

**I PRAY TO GOD, GODDESS,
THE ALL THAT IS,
THAT THIS BOOK WILL BE
THE BEGINNING OF THAT MOVEMENT.**

NOTES AND REFERENCES

[1] San Jose Mercury News: *Two Viruses Spreading Says Study,* Newsday, Sept. 14, 1990.

[2] *SE5 Biofield Research Manual,* Human Services Development Center, 1987, pg. II-5.

[3] Whitley Strieber, *Communion,* Avon, 1987.

[4] Valdamar Valerian, *Matrix II,* Leading Edge Research Group, Yelm, WA, 1990, pg 322.

[5] Roper Survey: *Unusual Personal Experiences,* Conducted for Bigelow Holding Co.,
The Roper Organization, Inc., NY, NY, 1991

[6] Contra Costa Times: *US Deliberately Released Radiation,* Melissa Healy, LA Times, Dec. 16, 1993.

[7] Time Magazine: *Death In The Mediterranean,* Nov. 12, 1990, Pg. 111.

[8] Marc Lappe, *Chemical Deception, The Toxic Threat to Health and the Environment,*
Sierra Club Books, 1992, pg. 84.

[9] Marc Lappe, Ibid., pg. 86.

[10] Marc Lappe, Ibid., pg. 86.

[11] San Francisco Chronicle, *Chemical Arms Pact Signed After 25 Years,* Norman Kempster,
LA Times, Jan. 4, 1993.

[12] Marc Lappe, Ibid., pg. 86.

[13] San Francisco Chronicle, *Study May Lead to new Alzheimer's Drugs,* Associated Press.

[14] Marc Lappe, Ibid., pg. 87.

[15] Marc Lappe, Ibid., pg. 88.

[16] Contra Costa Times: *Russia Reveals Chemical Worker Deaths,* Sergei Shargorodsky, Associated Press, Dec. 24, 1993.

[17] San Francisco Chronicle: *IBM Warns Workers on Chemicals and Miscarriages,* Staff, Wire Reports, Oct. 13, 1993.

[18] Honolulu Star-Bulletin, *Study of Women's Breast Cancer Finds a Link to PCB's, Pesticides,* Laurie Garrett, June 7, 1992.

[19] Contra Costa Times: *Full Transcripts of Oil Spill Tapes Ordered Released,* Rosanne Pagano,
Associated Press, Anchorage, Alaska

[20] Contra Costa Times: *Greek Tanker Spilled Nearly Twice As Much Oil as Exxon Valdez,* Associated Press, Dec. 14, 1992.

[21] Contra Costa Times: *Great Lakes Gunk is Toxic Puzzle for Region, Congress.* Katherine Rizzo, Associated Press, Dec. 13, 1993.

22 Marc Lappe, Ibid., pg. 80-89.

23 Marc Lappe, Ibid., pg. 83-84.

24 Seth Shulman, *The Threat At Home,* Beacon Press, 1992, pg. xiii.

25 San Francisco Examiner, *Toxic US Legacy in the Philippines,* Benjamin Pimentel and Louella J. Lasola, Special to Examiner.

26 Contra Costa Times: *Persian Gulf War Aftermath,* Joe Garofoli, Staff Writer, Dec. 12, 1993.

27 Seth Shulman, Ibid., pg. 28-30.

28 Seth Shulman, Ibid., pg. 27.

29 Seth Shulman, Ibid., pg. 28.

30 Seth Shulman, Ibid., pg. 29.

31 Seth Shulman, Ibid., general reading

32 Leon Chaitow, D.O., N.D. & Elizabeth Kutter, Ph.D., *How to Live with Low-Level Radiation,* Healing Arts Press, 1988, pg. 69-75. Steven R. Schechter, N.D., *Righting Radiation & Chemical Pollutants with Foods, Herbs & Vitamins,* Vitality, Inc., 1990, pg. 56-57.

33 San Francisco Chronicle: *Grim New Findings on Radiation Risks,* Matthew L. Ward, NY Times.

34 Contra Costa Times: *Russia Reveals Chemical Workers Deaths,* Sergei Shargorodsky, Associated Press, April 13, 1993, Contra Costa Times: *Pollution Ravages former USSR,* Donald M. Rothberg, Associated Press, April 13, 1992 Contra Costa Times: *This City Forgotten by God and Man,* Kathy Lally, Baltimore Sun.

35 San Francisco Chronicle: *U.S. Deliberately Released Radiation,* Melissa Healy, LA Times, Dec. 16, 1993,

36 Seth Shulman, Ibid., pg. 99.

37 San Francisco Chronicle: *Radioactive Soil Buried in Alaska,* Timothy Egan, NY Times.

38 GreenPeace Magazine: *Children of Chernoble,* Andre Carothers, Jan/Feb 1991.

39 San Francisco Chronicle: *U.S. Deliberately Released Radiation,* Melissa Healy, LA Times, Dec. 16, 1993

40 San Francisco Chronicle: *U.S. Deliberately Released Radiation,* Melissa Healy, LA Times, Dec. 16, 1993

41 Newsweek Magazine: *Chronic Fatigue Syndrome, A Modern Mystery,* Nov. 12, 1990, pg. 62

42 Contra Costa Times: *US Davis Pathologists Find Mysterious Virus That Kills Deer,* Marla Cone, LA Times, Dec. 8, 1993

43 Contra Costa Times: *Valley Fever Exploding Into Killer Epidemic,* Mark Orax, Dec. 23, 1992.

44 Contra Costa Times: *Babies Given Radiation, Report Says,* Gannett News Services, Dec. 1993.

45 San Francisco Chronicle: *Explosive Secret-Downed Jet Carried Atom Bomb,* Dan Reed, Chronicle Correspondent, Feb. 18, 1994.

46 San Francisco Chronicle: *AIDS-Like Virus in Cattle a Threat to Immune System,* Keith Schneider, NY Times, 1990.

47 Linda Moulton Howe: *An Alien Harvest,* Linda Moulton Howe Productions, Littleton, CO, 1989, pg. 110.

48 Cell Tech:, *General Information on Super Blue-Green Algae™ and Algae Products,* Klamath Falls, OR. Super Blue-Green Algae™ is a registered trademark of Cell Tech Corporation.

49 William H. Lee, R. Ph., Ph.D., *Coenzyme Q-10,* Keats Publishing, New Canaan, CN, 1987.

50 Dr. Glen Swartwout: *Electromagnetic Pollution Solutions,* Aerai Publishing, Hilo, HI, 1991.

51 *SE5 Biofield Research Manual,* Human Services Development Center, 1987,

52 Bob Fickes: *Ascension, The Time Has Come,* Council of Light, Inc. 1991, pg. 56-60.
Virginia Essene, Ed.: *New Cells, New Bodies, New Life!,* S.E.E. Publishing Co., Santa Clara, CA 1991, pg. 158-161.

53 Zacharia Sitchen: *The Wars of Gods and Men,* Avon Books, 1985, pg. 310.

54 David Hatcher Childress, *Vimana Aircraft of Ancient India & Atlantis Adventures Unlimited Press, 1991.*

APPENDIX 1

COMMON SYMPTOMS OF CHRONIC FATIGUE SYNDROME

More and more information seems to be coming to light concerning Chronic Fatigue Syndrome. Symptoms vary widely, and can come and go. Since symptoms can also be signs of other diseases, doctors commonly will diagnose CFIDS after all other possible disorders have been eliminated by blood tests and other diagnostic tools available to the medical profession. Estimates of the number of people who may be suffering from CFIDS disabilities in the US vary from 3 million to 10 million depending on how inclusive the definition and who is doing the estimating. A world-wide estimate of sufferers runs close to 90 million, and still counting. Many other countries such as Japan and Canada are taking this disease much more seriously than the US.

It is estimated that close to 70 percent of CFIDS sufferers are women. At least that was the case in the beginning. Statistics show that men are catching up rapidly, as are children, dogs, other pets, and cattle.

CENTER FOR DISEASE CONTROL DIAGNOSTIC CRITERIA FOR CHRONIC FATIGUE SYNDROME

Many people feel that our government has not done enough to validate the suffering and symptoms of those

183

with CFIDS. In fact, one gets the feeling that the government feels that if it ignores Chronic Fatigue Syndrome, the disorder will just disappear. I recently read in the newspaper that the CDC was in the process of redefining the criteria for diagnosis of Chronic Fatigue Syndrome. Under the new definition, the official number of cases would drop to about 300,000 sufferers. Now that really makes a whole lot of sense to me, just redefine the criteria and suddenly there are only a few people suffering from the symptoms! Do you get the impression that our government might be trying to cover-up this whole thing? I said it once before, and I will say it again: I seriously wonder if there is any connection between the symptoms of CFIDS and the secret nuclear program waged by our government that has just come to light. Only time will tell as the truth full comes to light.

I think it is important to take a look at the "official guidelines" developed by the CDC to determine if you or someone you know is suffering from Chronic Fatigue Syndrome.

MAJOR CRITERIA

1. New onset of fatigue lasting longer than six months with 50 percent reduction in activity.
2. No other medical or psychiatric conditions that could cause the symptoms.

MINOR CRITERIA

Symptoms must begin at or after onset of fatigue

1. Low-grade fever

2. Sore throat

3. Painful lymph nodes

4. Generalized muscle weakness

5. Muscle pain

6. Prolonged fatigue after exercise

7. Headaches

8. Joint pain

9. Sleep disturbance

10. Neuropsychologic complaints, such as forget-fulness, confusion, difficulty concentrating, de-pression.

11. Acute onset (over a few hours to a few days).

PHYSICAL CRITERIA

1. Low-grade fever

2. Throat inflammation

3. Palpable or tender lymph nodes

COMMON SYMPTOMS EXPERIENCED BY MANY CFIDS SUFFERERS

While no one denies that these symptoms are usually present, I personally feel the list needs to be expanded. Of a more realistic nature, I have put together a list of common symptoms experienced by myself and by others who suffer from CFIDS. I definitely feel that one of the major symptoms of CFIDS is the chronic yeast infections, and/or bacterial infections. Another criteria would be chronic food poisoning. Most people who suffer from this syndrome do not realize that they are subject to food poisoning.

COMMON REPORTED SYMPTOMS

1. Fatigue that is so overwhelming and devastating that it totally incapacitates the individual, draining every ounce of strength. I often used the analogy that it was like a battery that would not recharge. It only had so much energy. When it was depleted, it might take days or even weeks to recharge the battery.

2. Major symptoms developing over a few hours to a few days.

3. Symptoms triggered by emotional stress such as loss of loved one or job.

4. Symptoms triggered by illness or accident, including head injury, surgery, anesthesia, flu, mononucleosis.

5. Mild fever, chills

6. Sore throat, throat infections

7. Cough, Wheezing, Shortness of Breath

8. Development of Allergies including:
   - Sensitivity to household dust, molds
   - Intolerance for cigarette smoke
   - Sensitivity to inhalants and chemicals, including perfume
   - Allergies to foods not allergic to before onset
   - Allergies to medication, including penicillin drugs

9. Nasal Congestion, frequent sinus infections

10. Swollen or painful lymph nodes.

11. Generalized muscle weakness

12. Muscle soreness or discomfort

13. Prolonged fatigue following mild to moderate exercise

14. Joint pain without swelling or redness.

15. Numbness, tingling, burning sensations.

16. Skin rashes, hives, itching, burning or flushing of skin.

17. Sensitivity to bright sunlight

18. Frequent tearing or burning of eyes

19. Blind spots in visual field.

20. Irritability, tension, anxiety, hyperactivity, restlessness

21. Forgetfulness, confusion, difficulty thinking

22. Short term memory loss

23. Inability to focus and concentrate

24. Depression

25. Headaches

26. Unusual Brain Wave Patterns, Brain functioning in "Theta" rather than alert states of Alpha & Omega.

27. Disruption of electrical activity of brain as indicated by brain mapping.

28. Decreased Blood Flow to Brain as determined by testing.

29. Development of Dementia

30. Development of Brain Lesions (abnormal tissue)

31. Development of HTLV viruses causing Leukemia

32. Development of host of other viruses, including Herpes, Epstein Barr, Coxsackie, Mononucleosis, Hepatitis

33. Moderate to Severe Immune System Dysfunction
    - Imbalance In B-Cells
    - Imbalance in T-Cells
    - Imbalance in Phagocytic Cells
    - Imbalance in NK (Natural Killer) Cells

34. Development of Defective Red Blood Cells

35. Development of Chronic Systemic Candida Including:
    - Persistent and reoccurring vaginal discharge, itching, burning
    - Persistent abdominal bloating, pain, constipa-

tion, diarrhea, intestinal gas, and mucus in bowls.

36. Persistent Bad Breath, thick white coating of tongue

37. Broken Teeth

38. Bleeding Gums, mouth sores

39. Chronic Systemic Bacterial Infections Including:
    - Sinus Infections
    - Bladder/kidney infections
    - Vaginal and Urinary tract infections

40. Itching of Rectum

41. Food Poisoning

42. Craving for Sugar, Bread, or Alcoholic Beverage

43. Developing Intolerance for Alcohol

44. Developing Intolerance for Caffeine

45. Heartburn, Indigestion, Vomiting.

46. Ringing or Popping in Ears

47. Balance Disorders

48. Thyroid Imbalance

49. Adrenal Exhaustion, or Dysfunction

50. Endocrine System Imbalances

51. Back Pain in Kidney Area

52. Sleep Disorders including insomnia

53. Inability to access REM sleep state

54. Night Sweats

55. Nightmares

56. Swelling of Hands and Feet

57. Weight Loss

58. Weight Gain

59. Elevated Cholesterol

60. Intolerance to Cold

61. Changes in Menstrual Flow (profuse or extended menstrual bleeding)

62. Menstrual Dysfunction, Cramps, or PMS

63. Loss of Fingerprints

64. Disturbances in Rhythm and Speed of Heartbeat.

65. Calcium Deficiencies

66. Developing Bone Spurs on Spine, or fusion

67. Pin Point Pupils

68. Metabolism Imbalances

APPENDIX 2

The following is a list of Chronic Fatigue Organizations around the country. Most publish newsletters, and are there to provide information and help to people about Chronic Fatigue Syndrome.

NATIONAL CHRONIC FATIGUE SYNDROME ASSOCIATION
3521 Broadway, Suite 222
Kansas City, Missouri 64111
816.931.4777
****

CHRONIC FATIGUE IMMUNE DYSFUNCTION SYNDROME
ASSOCIATION
P.O. Box 220398
Charlotte, North Caroline 28222
800.44.CFIDS and 900 988-CFID
Marc Iverson, President
****

CHRONIC FATIGUE SYNDROME SOCIETY
P.O. Box 230108
Portland, Oregon 97223
503.684.5261
****

NATIONAL CHRONIC FATIGUE SYNDROME ADVISORY
COUNCIL
Corresponding Office: 12106 E. 54th Terrace
Kansas City, Missouri 64133
Dr. Anthony Komaroff, Council President

This organization of doctors, researchers and patients seeks to
improve access to accurate information about this disorder.
****

MINNAN, Inc.
P.O. Box 582
Glenview, Illinois 60025

Theodore Van Zeist, Director

This is a 30 year old private foundation, providing financial support to CFIDS research since 1984. It is also involved in keeping tract of federal developments related to CFS, and working with congressional appropriations committees.

****

CHRONIC FATIGUE IMMUNE DYSFUNCTION SYNDROME FOUNDATION
965 Mission St., Suite 425
San Francisco, California 94103
415.882.9986
Jan Montgomery, Director

Helps San Francisco public officials in tracking the incidence of chronic fatigue syndrome and gaining recognition for it as a public health priority.

UNITED FEDERATION OF CFS/CFIDS/CEBV ORGANIZATIONS
Box 14603
Tucson, Arizona 85732
602.298.8627
Larry A. Sakin, Chairman
An association helping to improve communication among patient support groups around the country.

****

CFIDS ACTION CAMPAIGN FOR THE UNITED STATES (CACTUS)
% CFIDS Foundation
965 Market Street, Suite 425
San Francisco, California 94103
415.882.9986

This organization is dedicated to raising public funds for support services and research, improved media coverage, and communication with other health organizations.

****

192

The Centers for Disease Control and the National Institutes of Health send free CFS information packets upon request.

CENTERS FOR DISEASE CONTROL
Attn: Josephine Lister
Bldg. 6 Room 121
Atlanta, Georgia 30333
404.639.1338
****

NATIONAL INSTITUTE OF ALLERGY AND INFECTIOUS DISEASES
Office of Communications
Bldg. 31 Room 7A-32
Bethesda, Maryland 20892
****

****

INTERNATIONAL CFS ORGANIZATIONS

Known as myalgic encephalomyelitis (ME) overseas, scientists have become increasingly certain that this is the same ailment. The largest organizations are the ME Society in England and ANZME Society in Australia and New Zealand.

AUSTRALIAN & NEW ZEALAND MYALGIC ENCEPHALOMYELITIS SOCIETY (ANZME)
P.O. Box 35-429
Browns Bay
Auckland 10, New Zealand
Contact: Jim Bookchurch
****

MYALGIC ENCEPHALOMYELITIS ASSOCIATION OF CANADA
1301 Plante Drive

Ottawa, Ontario, Canada
Contact: Rod Blaker
****

CANADA CFS INFORMATION
154 Timberline Trail
Aurora, Ontario L4G5Z5, Canada
Contact: Ann Teehan
****

MYALGIC ENCEPHALOMYELITIS ASSOCIATION
Box 8
Stanford-le-Hope
Essex SS17 8EX, England
Contact: Peter M. Blackman
****

DUTCH MYALGIC ENCEPHALOMYELITIS FOUNDATION
M.E. Stichting
Postbus 23670
11000ED Amsterdam ZO, Holland
Contact: Marion Lescrauwaet
****

HONG KONG ME INFORMATION
60B Conduit Road, 3rd Floor
Hong Kong
Contact: D. Edwards
****

PAPAU, NEW GUINEA MYALGIC ENCEPHALOMYELITIS
SUPPORT
Box 44
Ukarumpa, Via Lac, Papua, New Guinea
****

ME AWARENESS GROUP
66 Third Street
Lower Houghton, 2198 South Africa
Contact: Janine Shawell
****

APPENDIX 3

Recommended Reading List
Books on Chronic Fatigue Syndrome

CFIDS: The Disease of a Thousand Names. By Dr. David S. Bell, Pollard Publications. 1991.
Discussion of syndrome, including technical explanation of the mechanisms thought by the author to cause it.

What Really Killed Gilda Radner? Frontline Reports on the CFS Epidemic. By Neenyah Ostrom. That New Magazine Inc. 1991.
This New York Native writer looks at the politics behind Chronic Fatigue Syndrome.

CFIDS: An Owner's Manual by Barbara Brooks and Nancy Smith. 1988. (Available from Barbara Books & Nancy Smith, Box 6456, Silver Springs, Maryland 20906.)
This handbook is written and self-published by two CFIDS patients. It focuses on the debilitating social and emotional consequences of the illness and how to cope with them.

Chronic Fatigue & Tiredness. By Susan M. Lark, M.D. Westchester Publishing Company. 1993.
A Self-Help Program offering effective solutions for conditions associated with Chronic Fatigue Syndrome, candida, allergies, PMS, menopause, anemia, low thyroid, and depression.

Chronic Fatigue Syndrome: A Personal Diary. By Arnold H. Goldberg, M.D. (Available from Dr. A.H. Goldberg, 920 King St. West, Kitchener, Ontario, Canada N2G 1G4.)
This spiral-bound workbook is designed to let sufferers keep records of their medical history, including visits to physicians, and to monitor treatment and medications received. Designed to facilitate daily entries.

The Mile High Staircase. By Toni Jeffreys. Hodder and Stoughton, 1982. (Available from ANZME, P.O. Box 35-429, Browns Bay Auckland 10, New Zealand)
Australian women tell of their struggle with Chronic Fatigue Syndrome. A very moving story.

Chronic Fatigue Syndrome: A Victim's Guide to Understanding, Treating, And Coping with This Debilitating Illness. By Gregg Charles Fisher. Warner Books, 1989.
This is a personal story of a young divinity student and his wife who have been incapacitated by this disease for at least ten years.

Hope And Help For Chronic Fatigue Syndrome. By Karyn Feiden. Simon & Schuster, 1990.
The author considers this book an official guide of the CFS/CFIDS Network, and offers a practical approach to overcoming CFIDS.

Chronic Fatigue Syndrome: The Hidden Epidemic. By Jesse Stoff, M.D. and Charles Pellegrino. Random House, 1988.
A doctor writes about his approach to treatment of CFIDS patients. He strongly feels that liver-related problems are the underlying source of the syndrome.

50 Things You Should Know About the Chronic Fatigue Syndrome Epidemic. By Neenyah Ostrom. St. Martin's Paperback, 1993.
Author probes the facts and answers questions about CFIDS in this easy to read look at the disease.

Social Security Benefits and Chronic Fatigue Syndrome. By Samuel J. Imperati and Janis Pearson. (Available from CFIDS Society, Box 230108, Portland Oregon 97223.)
Written specifically for CFIDS patients, this booklet gives important information for obtaining Social Security disability benefits.

Social Security Disability Benefits: How to Get Them! How To Keep Them! By James W. Ross. (Available from Ross Publishing Co., 188 Forrester Rd., Slippery Rock, Pennsylvania 16075, or the CFIDS Society, Box 230108, Portland, Oregon 97223.)
More information about applying for Social Security Benefits.

Books on Toxic Substances

Chemical Deception, The Toxic Threat To Health and The Environment. By Marc Lappe. Sierra Club Books, 1991.
In this book Lappe exposes ten key myths about toxic chemicals that endanger us all, and effect our health on this planet.

The Threat At Home, Confronting The Toxic Legacy Of The U.S. Military. By Seth Shulman. Beacon Press, 1992.
Shulman exposes the dangers posed to the public by toxic substances that saturate most military bases and installations around the US. This book is the first comprehensive account of the US military's history of toxic waste production and dumping, and the environmental implications to citizens.

Electromagnetic Pollution Solutions, By Dr. Glen Swartwout. Aerai Press, 1991. Covers the scope of electromagnetic stress-related illness. Discusses the source of stress, how they affect you and your family.

How To Live with Low-Level Radiation, by Ceon Chaitow, D.O., N.D. & Elizabeth Kutter, Ph.D., Healing Arts Press, 1988.

Fighting Radiation & Chemical Pollutants With Food, Herbs, & Vitamins, by Steven R. Schechter, N.D. Vitality, Ink, 1990.

Books on Vibrational Healing

Vibrational Medicine. By Richard Gerber, M.D., Bear & Co., 1988. This comprehensive book covers the subjects of energetic medicine, including homeopathic remedies, flower essences, crystal healing, therapeutic though, acupuncture, radionics, electrotherapy, herbal medicine, psychic healing, and therapeutic radiology. This book covers theory, history and spiritual philosophy.

Channeled Books

New Cells, New Bodies, New Life, by Virginia Essene, ed., S.E.E. Publishing Co. 1991.
Channeled information about our earth in transition and the state of human health. Looks at the possibility that we are undergoing massive cellular changes from the dense matter we find ourselves housed in today. Looks at influence of past lives in DNA.

Ascension, The Time is Now, by Bob Fickes, Council of Light, Inc., 1991.
Channeled information from Ascended Masters concerning changes in humans as the vibrations raise on earth.

Books on the History of Earth

Vimana Aircraft of Ancient India & Atlantis, By David Childress, Adventures Unlimited Press, 1991.
Information based on Ancient Indian texts, Ramayana and Mahabharata, are used to prove existence of aircraft more than 4000 years ago. Included are information about Rama Empire and the wars that destroyed it during Atlantian times.

The Wars Of Gods and Men, by Zacharia Sitchen, Avon Books, 1985.

The 12th Planet, by Zacharia Sitchen, Avon Books, 1985.

The Stairway to Heaven, by Zacharia Sitchen, Avon Books.

INDEX

from third world, 118
steamed, 137
vegetables, fresh, 137
verbal ability, impaired, 73
Veterans Affairs Agency,
83
**Viamana Aircraft of
Ancient India and
Atlantis,** 168
vibrations, lowered, 164
violence, gods, 171
violence near military
bases or chemical
plants, 86
viral & immune system
diseases, all same
disease, 124
viruses, 27
and extraterrestrials, 64
grow on toxic chemicals
and radioactive sub-
stances, 113
homeopathic remedies
for, 145
mutations, 56
overgrowth, 113
search for, 53-59
in subtle bodies, 55
visual space organization
problems, 73
Vitamin K, 144
vitamins, 43, 135, 140
Vitrons, 52
volcanoes, people sacri-
ficed to, 174-175

voltage, increased, 62-63
vomiting, 73, 76
vows of "undying love"
and soul fusion, 175

–W–

war
contamination source,
119
versus human life,
relative importance of,
127
**Wars Between Gods
and Men,** 168
Washington, 93, 95
waste oils, 87
water
buying purified, 134
contaminated, 66, 96,
98, 119-120
drinking at restaurants,
135
irrigation, 92
near military or indus-
trial area, 135
purifying, 134-135
radioactive contamina-
tion in, 105
source, Western states,
93
tap, 44, 134
toxic chemical residues
in, 45
water purifier, 45
weight loss, 81

Address:_____

_____

Date: _____

Senator John Glenn, D-Ohio
Chairman
Committee on Government Affairs
US. Senate
Washington, D. C. 20510

Re: Secret Nuclear Weapons Research Program

Dear Senator Glenn:

I have recently become aware of your interest in our government's Secret Military Nuclear Research Program. Like all citizens, I am alarmed and concerned about the unauthorized use and testing of radioactive materials.

I am concerned about the rights of citizens of the United States, guaranteed by our Constitution, being violated. I wonder just how many people have been involved in research without their knowledge or consent. I am also concerned about radioactive fallout contaminating our food and water supplies.

I support your efforts in this matter. I encourage you to keep this investigation going until all has been revealed to the citizens of the US. You have my support to keep uncovering information until the full extent of damage is known. It is of utmost importance that all steps are taken to remedy the situation.

I want to know if I, or my loved ones have been victims of this program. I want to know if Chronic Fatigue Syndrome and other forms of cancer and immune dysfunction disease are the result of a massive nuclear research program and the resulting nuclear waste.

Sincerely,

_____(signature)

_____(Print name)

We Need Your Help
Money Is Needed
To Help CFIDS Sufferers

Money is desperately needed to help people suffering from Chronic Fatigue Syndrome and other immune dysfunction diseases who have no money for treatment.

Few people who suffer from Chronic Fatigue Syndrome have a job or other source of income. Many are forced into bankruptcy. Most do not have money for treatment. Many can be helped to turn the corner and regain their health.

Your tax deductible gift can help a great deal. If you feel that my information has value and can help others, please look into your heart and send us your donation today.

Thank you and may God/Goddess Bless You.

Suzann Marie Angelus

· ·

Yes, I want to help. Please find enclosed my tax-deductible gift in the amount of $_____.

Make check payable to: Reunion Center of Light

Name: _____

Address: _____

_____

Phone: (_____ _____

Mail to: Suzann Marie Angelus, c/o Reunion Center of Light, 140 Mayhew Way, Suite 202, Pleasant Hill, CA 94523

For Information, Call: 510/631-0360

Order Form

We hope you have found the information in this book helpful. If you would like to order additional copies, please ask for it at your local bookstore. If it is unavailable, you may order it directly by using the order form below.

Item	Qty	Price Ea	Total
CFS, Aids & Immune Dysfunction Disease, The Cause & the Cure		$15.95	
Polarizers for ELF Waves		$75	

Shipping & Handling	Subtotal	

Merchandise Subtotal	Add	Shipping & Handling	
under $20	3.00		
$20-$40	5.00	Sales Tax (CA residents add 8.25%)	
$40-$75	7.00		
$75-$100	9.00		
over $100	10% of total		
Allow 3-4 weeks for delivery		Total Enclosed	

Name _____

Address _____

_____
City   State   Zip

MAIL TO:
Symbolic Productions, PO Box 6705, Moraga, CA 94556
For information, call: 510/631-0360

Please send me information on the following products

I am interested in:

Super Blue-Green Algae™

☐ Products

☐ Wholesale Purchases

☐ Distributor

Magnets

☐ Information on magnets

SE5 Biofield Spectrum Analyzer

☐ Information on SE5

Hair Analysis

☐ Information on Hair Analysis with SE5

Name _____

Address _____

City   State   Zip

MAIL TO:
Symbolic Productions, PO Box 6705, Moraga, CA 94556